Wrestling
with the
Angel

Conscious Living, Loving and Dying

River King

The poem on page 7 is an excerpt from Der Schauende by Rainer Maria Rilke, translated by
Christine Cooke and River King.

Matador
9 Priory Business Park,
Wistow Road, Kibworth Beauchamp,
Leicestershire. LE8 0RX
Tel: 0116 279 2299
Email: books@troubador.co.uk
Web: www.troubador.co.uk/matador
Twitter: @matadorbooks

ISBN 978 1785893 063

British Library Cataloguing in Publication Data.
A catalogue record for this book is available from the British Library.

Typeset in 11.5pt Baskerville by Troubador Publishing Ltd, Leicester, UK

Matador is an imprint of Troubador Publishing Ltd

Amanda

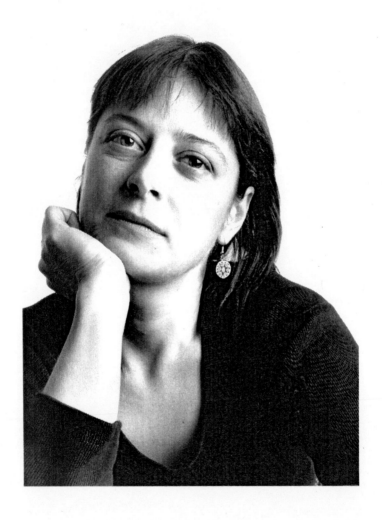

Don't be discouraged by your incapacity to dispel darkness from the world. Light your candle and step forward.

Mata Amritanandamayi Devi

What we choose to fight is so small
And success diminishes us.
What will not be bent by us
Is The Eternal and The Immense.

That is the Angel who appeared
To the wrestlers in the Old Testament:
When his opponents' sinews
Stretched like metal strings,
He felt them beneath his fingers
Like chords of deep melodies.

Whoever this Angel overcame, who
So often refrained from fighting,
Left those all powerful hands, reformed
Devout and comforted and great.

Victory does not entice this man.
His growth is in
Being deep-defeated
By ever greater beings.

FOREWORD

Love is an Angel that heals and inspires. Leukaemia is one of those 'ever greater beings that enfold and reform us through deep defeat.'

Close relationships offer us the opportunity to develop towards conscious being. Learning to live together, to accept the other's reality and perceptions while staying true to our own selves requires a high level of openness and honesty.

Living with a life-threatening disease raises the stakes for both partners. Illness can be a powerful catalyst to accelerate the process of inner change, but it can also bring it to a numbing standstill. The person who has the illness may have pressing physical needs that demand immediate attention so deeper matters are left aside.

It doesn't have to be like that. With the help of greater consciousness it is possible to create and live meaningful lives while going through difficult times.

This is the story of how Amanda and I lived and loved each other through her illness. By the time we met she had been dealing with leukaemia for eight years and had found her own unique way to respond to it, seeing herself as a sensitive and intelligent woman living with a life-threatening illness rather than just as a helpless victim. I had never been really ill nor close to someone with such an illness and had no idea of how this would affect me.

Serious illness is more than just a body problem. It affects our deepest inner processes, our hearts and minds, and this is where healing and transformation can take place. For healing does not mean a return to the state we were in before, rather it requires that we move on to somewhere completely new, to a place of inner wholeness that is reflected out towards the world. This is true for the lover and carer as well as for the one afflicted.

A life-threatening disease wakes us up to the knowledge that our time here is limited. It makes us ask the big questions about life. We have to think about how we are to live, not just in the sense of home and work, but about our real purpose in life and the deeper significance of our presence on earth. We don't wish to die saying, "What was the point of all that?"

And death itself is rarely discussed. There is such fear of dying that people avoid the subject despite it being the one event that is common to every life. While we cannot know what comes after death, we can learn to live with awareness of our mortality, knowing that we could die tomorrow or live for many years to come.

Amanda and I tried to live authentically as our essential selves and characters. Our story shows how consciously facing our difficulties and talking about what was going on helped us to live in ways that were meaningful to us.

In the process we were both profoundly changed.

Part One

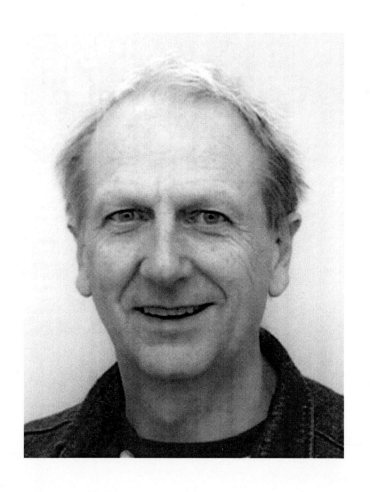

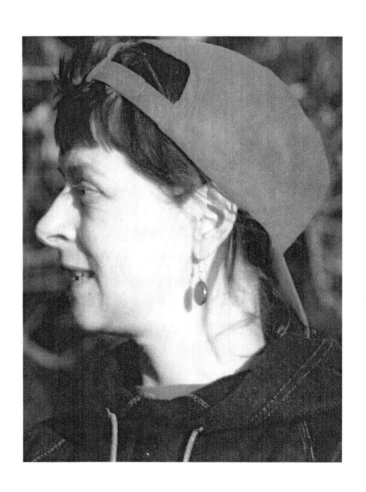

1

It was in the middle of the second day that I found myself rolling on the floor, laughter bubbling up from my belly and through my body in a way I had never felt before. This was ecstasy.

I was on a weekend course in improvisation and the art of clowning. Lex, our teacher, explained, "This sort of clowning means being your true and sensitive self, not trying to be funny or clever. It's not circus clowning. In the workshop we will explore spontaneity through movement, dance and song without the use of words. If this brings up laughter then let yourself laugh, if it brings tears then let yourself cry. There are no big explanations, no erudite teaching, it is learning through experience."

I found his talk exciting. I liked the idea of really being my true and authentic self, instead of just talking about it as I had in the past.

"Take off your mask and be yourself," he said. And I had imagined that being a clown meant putting on a mask.

"Don't think about it, don't try to understand it. All you have to do is to stop thinking and follow your intuition."

I decided to trust him. As I got into it I relaxed and gave myself over to the exercises. I began to enjoy myself in ways I had not done since I was a child, without feeling I was being childish. As well as moving and dancing with others I was laughing and singing. This was not how I normally behaved, and I loved it.

I realised that until then my laughing had always been in my throat, usually in response to a joke, a cartoon or comedy. This time no-one was trying to be funny and yet I was laughing. Laughing with my whole body, with joy and relief at the open and simple ways we were all relating to each other, just as Lex had said, without any talking. With his guidance and our spontaneity we had created an atmosphere of warmth and trust, lightly touched by moments of humour.

I was begiunning to learn about improvisation, being in a situation where you don't know what is going to happen and don't know what you are going to do. You have no opportunity to try and work things out. You cannot think, you simply have to allow your intuition to be your guide. The results were always unexpected and sometimes incredibly funny.

By the end of the weekend I'd had a taste of a different way to be myself. I found it strange to be so open and imaginative. It was as if a whole new side of my character was opening up. And I liked it

Six weeks later I went on another weekend with Lex and after that a week-long course. I loved what I was learning and the people I was meeting. At the end of it Lex told us he would be starting a three-year part time training in the autumn.

I wanted to do it but wondered about making such a big commitment and having to find so much money to pay for it all.

It was a difficult time in my life. I was living with my wife in our shared home but our marriage was in dire straits and I didn't know how much longer it would survive. As well as that I was feeling frustrated and unsatisfied in my work.

Then one night I had a startling dream that woke me up in shock. I was being interviewed by my boss for the job I was already doing. I didn't get the job and my boss said, "Nick, you have no future in Further Education. You have to find another way." I woke up panicking about how I would earn my living. Generally I believe that dreams have something important to say to me, and this one was unusually explicit. As the day went by I thought about its meaning and eventually realised it revealed what I had not wanted to admit. It was telling me that I was really struggling and could not carry on in this kind of work. For the sake of my mental health I would need to quit and look for something else.

The idea filled me with alarm as no alternative came to mind. But unknown to me fate had already started things moving. A few months later I was told there was to be a big reorganisation of the college, and that if I wished I could apply for voluntary redundancy. Within a year I would be offered a good financial deal and then be free.

Soon to be single, solvent and fifty years old, with no plans or employment prospects, I began to wonder about my future. I did not want a repeat of all mistakes I had made in the past. Perhaps the Art of Clowning would feature in some way, would lead me on to a completely different and more authentic way of living. Maybe Lex's three year training would be the opening I needed.

2

I made a new circle of friends in the first year of the training. We were all on an unknown path together, exploring where this clowning would take us. With Lex's guidance we opened our hearts and minds to intuition, spontaneity and creativity. We played, moved, danced and made music, enjoying ourselves without the use of words or rational thinking. We improvised scenes and acts together and experimented with creating costumes and putting on make up. We learned to speak jabber talk, that nonsense language where meaning comes from intonation and gesture. By the end of each of these training weeks I felt a greater sense of myself as a creative being with more potential than I ever imagined.

As part of the clown training we often worked in pairs and small groups to create acts that we then performed for the others. One of the clowns, Amanda, wrote a description of an act that she and I had created together:

> *There are two clowns on the stage, but each appears unaware of the other. One holds a red rose, the other a pink one. Each clown gazes out at the audience as if searching for a long lost friend. They look so lonely and the plaintive music seems to emphasise their sadness. Their search for love grows more desperate, they look everywhere, behind curtains, under*

chairs, up in the air, but love is not found. Eventually, as if by chance, they are standing next to each other, each lost in his own world. Yet although their eyes do not meet, their hands move towards each other and they swap the flowers they hold. Each marvelling at his new flower, the clowns wander off in opposite directions, still not realising that the other was so close, searching for the same thing.

The audience laughs, but with recognition and compassion for the all-too-human predicament. The clowns showed the sadness of being lonely and lost in one's own pre-occupations. Yet they shared their flowers, penetrating the thin veil that hid them from true contact. For those two clowns this was not a made-up story. It came from genuine sadness about not being able to find true love. As clowns they were able to put real feelings into a symbolic form that was touching, playful and humorous. Their apparent blindness in not seeing each other mirrors many situations in life; we often do not realise that the abundance we seek is all around us.

It was an act we were to perform together in public several times in the future.

Our training with Lex took place in a residential centre so there was plenty of time to meet and talk over meals and free time. Groups of us would go for walks in nature, go down to the sea for a swim or share a beer at the local pub. Over the months I formed good friendships with Val, Phil, Carola, Jenny, and got on well with the others. But it was Amanda with whom I had the greatest affinity and we often talked together.

In the spring holiday that year I was staying with friends in south Devon and rang Amanda who lived in the north of the county to suggest I go over to visit her.

I drove across Dartmoor through thick black clouds, strong winds and heavy rain. It was hard going, further than I had imagined, and I was wondering if it was worth the effort. Then I came over the top of a hill and was met by an astonishing sight. A wide valley opened up below me lit by brilliant rays of sunshine flooding through a gap in the threatening skies. A bright and vivid double rainbow arched across the valley complete from end to end, the most intense colours I had ever seen. I stopped to watch, the rain still drumming on the roof of the car, and sat for five minutes with a sense of awe and joy. I had the feeling that the world was giving me a sign of hope, that whatever difficulties I might have to face just now, there was a bright and shining future to be found ahead of me.

I arrived in time for us to have cream tea in a cafe and then later supper at a hotel down by the edge of the sea. I told her about the rainbow and how it seemed to symbolise my current life situation, and gave her a bare outline of what I was living through and how my future was so unknown.

She told me she had been living and working in India for some time but had returned to England for health reasons. She felt she was lucky to find a job as house manager in a residential centre, though it was not all easy going. Her employers, she said, were quite unusual people who lived their lives according to the promptings of their spirit guides. They made their decisions by dowsing for advice according to the swinging of a pendulum and she never knew what they would come up with next.

The following day was sunny and warm so we went for a walk along the cliffs and by the sea, enjoying our time together. My emotions were in turmoil, finding myself taking such delight in her company and feeling drawn to get closer, yet not wanting to make my life any more complicated. I said nothing of my thoughts and feelings and neither did she.

3

It was in June that my unhappy marriage finally came to an end and I left my home for the last time. I went down the drive feeling a surge of excitement as the weight of all the stress and struggles fell away. I felt light and free, taking none of my possessions other than my car and a few clothes.

Clown-like, I had no plans. A friend had said I could stay in his spare bedroom for a couple of weeks but beyond that I had not wanted to arrange anything. I had given no thought to the future.

And then came a simple phone call from my friend David, "Katy and I will be away for six weeks, would you like to house sit for us?" Life seemed to be taking care of me.

I loved their house with its large rooms and light windows, the feeling of space and beauty. I felt refreshed by Katy's artistic creations and flower decorations. It was perfect to stop and rest on the lawn in the walled garden with flowers all around me in the late June warmth and summer evenings. I needed this space to recover after all the turmoil.

I tried not to think about what I had left behind, enjoying my easy freedom to do and be as I pleased. I lay in bed listening to the morning birds, went walking in the Chiltern Hills, borrowed David's bike and rode out along the old railway track. I drove in to Oxford and wandered the narrow lanes, admiring the old sandstone university buildings, drank coffee in Blackwells, leafing through books borrowed from the shelves.

I enjoyed the space, living alone with no responsibilities. I meditated in the dawn sunlight, sat in the garden, ate mangoes for breakfast, walked in the woods with a picnic of French bread, tomatoes and Italian salami. I picked books from the long shelves on the landing and read late into the night.

One weekend I had a clown gathering to go to which I knew would be light and supportive. Before going I re-read the piece Amanda had written and shared with us at our last meeting:

> *At the core of sacred clowning is the sense that each person is part of something greater, a source of being which connects with everything. Each creative act brings the sacred clown to a moment of surrender to mystery. He does not know what will happen next. He plays on the edge between the familiar world and the vastness of the cosmos.*

Yes. That was where I was. Playing on the edge between the safety of the familiar and the unknown realms of possibility. I was done with my old conventional life and ready for a new experience of living.

Waking from my reverie I prepared for the weekend ahead. We all met at the usual hall, Val, Carola, Didier, Amanda,

Jenny, Arno, Phil, Susan and the others. I felt easy and relaxed with them, all sitting in a circle on the floor, each one talking about how their lives and clown practice had gone over the last months.

When it came to my turn I told them that I had finally left my home and was living with friends for a while. Several people said they thought this was a positive step for me and wished me well. When it was Amanda's turn to speak she said she had been asked to leave her job and flat in Devon at short notice. It seemed that her employers had consulted their spirit advisers again and the pendulum had swung indicating that they should change the direction of their business. As a result they said they wanted Amanda to leave and find somewhere else to live. As it was at such short notice she had gone to stay with an old friend in Oxford.

Oxford! So near to where I was staying. My heart leapt. Fate, life and the swing of the pendulum were pushing us closer in the most unexpected way. After the weekend it was natural for us to meet up in town and go for walks and meals together.

It was on one of these outings that Amanda asked if I would help her put on a performance in October in Brixton where she used to live. As part of our clown training Lex had asked us each to find a venue, get an audience and put on a clown show. This would be our first attempt at going public without the whole group together. I agreed at once and we arranged to meet often to create a show, to find music and make costumes. It would be at the Brixton Cancer centre. She explained that she had health problems and the people there had been very helpful to her in the past. She didn't dwell on the subject and I didn't want to intrude upon her private life.

As the weeks went by, long warm sunny evenings, we saw more of each other. In the quiet times between our meetings I sat in the garden and wondered what was going on between us, these unexpected feelings I had, the warmth in my heart, the physical longing. Was I sliding unawarely into a new relationship, so soon after leaving the last? Surely that would be totally irresponsible. But the feelings were mutual. Amanda told me she had felt attracted to me for a long time but held back while I was still in my marriage. Hearing her say this I lost all sense of myself and my mind ceased to function. I just wanted us to merge together in a warm and passionate bundle of loving. But at other times we talked sensibly, discussed the realities. One of these was her health, or lack of it. She told me that she had a form of leukaemia which might shorten her life. I didn't ask her any more, not wanting to know the details because I was so deep in the romance.

Summer rolled on. David and Katy came back from their holiday and said I could stay on with them for a few more weeks until the end of August. I was happy to accept, it was easy living with them. They were giving me time to sort out my head and begin to think more seriously about my future. I knew I would have to leave sometime but found it hard to imagine where to go next. With no aims or ambitions, I simply wanted to take it easy for a while longer.

Amanda was in a similar situation and told me she couldn't stay with her friends for much longer either.

One evening she and I were sitting in the back garden enjoying the evening sun, before going into town to get a pizza for supper. We were wondering about our future and I made what seemed to be an obvious suggestion: "Look, we both need to find somewhere to live. Why don't we think of finding a place to share?"

"That would be a big step for us," Amanda replied. "And before we get too serious you need to know a bit more about me and what you might be letting yourself in for. Let's talk about it in the car."

4

In the car park she turned to me.

"You do know I have leukaemia, don't you?"

"Yes, you did tell me."

"Do you know anything about it, what it means?"

"To be honest, I know almost nothing."

"Not many people do. But as we are thinking of getting together I need you to know what life with leukaemia is like and how things may change for me as time goes on. I don't usually tell people about this as I find their responses too difficult. They are either cloyingly sympathetic or else embarrassed and begin to avoid me."

She paused and looked searchingly into my face. "I want to share this with you so you understand where I am coming from."

"That seems a good idea. But is this the best place to talk?"

"Here is as good as anywhere, and the time feels right. Listen. What I have is called Chronic Myeloid Leukaemia. It's a form of cancer, cancer of the blood. Most people die a year or two after diagnosis. I am very unusual in that I've had it for eight years. I've survived mainly because of the amazing help from the oncologists at St Thomas' hospital in London."

"Oh" I said, not knowing what else to say.

"I've had a lot of treatments, including chemotherapy and what is called an autologous bone marrow transplant. I spent six weeks in an isolation ward as any infection could have been the end of me. Now my health is very variable. I go up and down, sometimes feeling really weak and ill. If I get a cold it is much worse for me than for a healthy person. I take a plateful of drugs every day and have to go to the hospital in London quite often to see the specialists."

"I see. I didn't know." I sat silent, listening as she went on.

"According to the statistics my future is quite predictable, only the timing is unknown. What usually happens is that at some stage the leukaemia turns from being chronic to being acute. Then everything gets worse and over a period of six months the patient gradually goes downhill, gets weaker, more vulnerable and eventually dies."

We were both silent. I felt a deep sinking in my guts, and tears itching in the corners of my eyes.

"But that is just the statistics. It's only a probability. My position may be right at the edge of the probability curve. No-one can actually predict my future, and I may be a rare exception. I may have many years to live and have not given up hope for a miracle recovery. And I'm not asking for sympathy, I'm only telling you because I think you need to know. I would rather you knew it all now, and made a conscious decision about whether you really want to get closer. I would hate to have you stay a while and then leave because it is too much. My last boyfriend decided he couldn't cope with it all and we parted. That was painful, but at least he was honest about it."

"I don't know what to say. I don't know what I feel, except surprised, shocked, sad and confused."

"You don't have to decide anything right now. Take your time and ask whatever you want."

This was so sudden and unexpected, far beyond anything I had experienced, beyond anything I had ever imagined. I needed space to collect my thoughts before we talked more. We got out of the car and instead of heading for the High Street we turned towards the park and walked in silence under the trees beside the river. It was some time before I was able to talk, and even longer before I could think of eating.

Eventually hunger called and we found a Pizza Express that was not too busy and a quiet table in the corner. We ordered food and a glass of red wine, and returned to our conversation.

"I've lived with it for a long time now," she said, "and I want to tell you more of my thoughts and feelings, so you understand how I deal with it. I don't want any misunderstandings."

"Go on, I want to hear."

"I hate it when people refer to leukaemia as a terminal illness, and act as if I will soon be dead. I call it a life-threatening illness and think of myself and describe myself as living. I emphasise I am living. I am not dying. Dying is something that may come at some time in the future, but I am not dying now. I am living with difficult symptoms and want to be seen as such, not as a sick patient who has no mind of her own and should be handled with kid gloves. While I may at times feel weak, fearful and vulnerable, underneath all that I am myself, a living, loving human being. Don't ever forget that, even when I'm lying on my death bed."

We talked some more, and then agreed to leave it there, to give me time to think, to take it all in. I dropped her off at her friend's house and drove back to David's.

5

This was shocking and unexpected. I was stunned at the enormity of her symptoms, moved by her honesty and deeply impressed at the way she had come to live with the realities she was facing. But did I really want to get more involved with her, to get closer and then have to deal with her illness if things got worse?

I had to think about myself and my future. What did I want to do with my life? I had only just left a twenty-year marriage and was certainly not ready to embark on a new relationship. I needed to sort myself out, find a new direction in life and a place to live. I had not really meant to suggest we have a relationship; my idea had been just to rent a place to share for a while. This was so much more.

But I was drawn to her, perhaps in love. I had forgotten what new love felt like, and this was very powerful. During the clown training we had spent many hours together and something about her had touched my heart. I felt she had found a way to live her life that was truly authentic, based on an honest recognition of who she was. That was a complete contrast to how my previous married life had been.

We didn't meet for a few days and I had several sleepless

nights, thoughts whirling in my head, turning restlessly. What should I do? I wasn't ready for this. I had enough to deal with sorting out my own life. I needed more time to get my head clear. It was all too much to take in and I reached a stage where I just didn't want to think about it any more, didn't want to look at what was going on. I just wanted to have a bit of space and fall asleep. But that seemed impossible.

On one of those nights when I thought I would never sleep I must have drifted off. And then, in a mix of dreams and drowsy thoughts, I was suddenly fully awake. I heard a voice calling to me. It was a clear and striking voice, speaking with wisdom and authority.

"This is your role for the coming years. To help her and support her whatever comes. And you will receive more than you give. You will be transformed. This is the spiritual journey you are offered."

It was as if someone was standing in the room speaking to me though there was no-one to see. There was total certainty in the voice and the message was clear but its content was quite unexpected. This would be a spiritual journey, I would receive more than I would give and I would be transformed.

I was shocked into being fully awake. Had I been dreaming? Where did this come from? Who was speaking? Was it just a dream? Did it come from my unconscious or from somewhere outside?

This message was so totally different from anything I had thought before. While I had wondered if I could cope with her being ill I had never thought about how I might be affected on a deeper level. And now here was the idea that I would be changed in deep and significant ways.

I lay there, awake in the night, wondering where my life was to go, what direction I should take. It was such an extraordinary thing to hear. I thought back to other dreams I'd had in the past, ones that had helped me clarify where I was in my life. Now here was a new one that could not be ignored. I was being given a choice and I felt I was free to choose, could accept or reject, and yet it was made very clear which path would be the one for me to take. It would lead me to an inner transformation.

Morning came and I tried to look at it all in an objective manner. Rationally I knew this was all too soon, too sudden, that I was not ready for it, needed time. But I could not ignore the dream. On a deeper level inside I knew I would say yes, would go forward into whatever was to come. Even though my mind said don't rush into it, I understood this was to be my future. And deep inside I felt a surge of joy that I would step out of my old way of life into this journey of love. Deep down I was aware I needed nothing less than the total transformation that I was being offered.

6

The following day we arranged to meet and go for a walk down by the river. She listened as I recounted my dream and how I had been so surprised. I went on to tell her about all my thoughts and feelings.

"So you see, that's where I am. I am taking it as a message from my higher self telling me clearly what is going on. I find it amazing to be so sure that this is what I should do. And amazing to be saying this directly to your face. You, and the clowning, are helping me to open up. What this really means is that I am ready to explore and live our lives together, and that I will deal with whatever comes up as best I can. We are bound to have different hopes and expectations, and leukaemia will add its own special challenges."

She smiled, a bloom of joy spreading out across her face, and said, "That makes me very happy. And I am so glad you are doing this for yourself, not out of some sense of pity for my situation. It gives me hope that we can have a good and honest relationship."

We went on to talk about how we might go forward, what sort of place we would want to rent, and where. She knew and liked the area known as East Oxford, not too far from the centre of town nor from the river. So that was where we would begin our search. We decided to start visiting estate agents the next week.

After that we got together often, learnt more about each other and grew closer. I was moved by the quality of our relationship and the openness and honesty in the way she lived and expressed her feelings. I tried to match her, but still found it hard to be so open and un-guarded.

"I'm quite a private sort of person and don't find it easy to talk about my feelings. I grew up in a very male environment and we just didn't do that sort of thing. I lived with my parents and two older brothers and went to all boys schools. My mother was almost the only woman in my life until I started dating girls. Then I got married in my early twenties and even there we didn't talk much about feelings or deeper thoughts. It just wasn't something I ever did."

"That's a fairly typical male experience. Men seldom talk about their emotions and personal thoughts."

"Well, I'm trying now. It's only because of the co-counselling and other courses I did that I even know what feelings really are. And if my life hadn't been falling apart I would never have dreamed of getting help and doing any of those sorts of things. Up until then I preferred to be thinking and doing things, rather than exploring my feelings"

"Yes, that's like most of the men I know."

"And I don't have much experience of being ill. The worst was when I had the awful pain of a slipped disc followed by six weeks on my back. But I recovered from that with no permanent damage.

"So what was it like to discover you had leukaemia? I have no idea how I would react if told I had cancer."

Our pace slowed, we stopped to watch a swan drifting on the water, then found a patch of short grass and sat on the riverbank.

"It was back in 1984 when I was twenty seven, working in an office at a rather ordinary secretarial job. I shared a flat in Brixton with another woman and we had a pretty good social life. I had been feeling weak for ages and finally went to see the doctor about my swollen stomach and immense tiredness. The results of the blood tests came back very quickly and I was called back to the surgery. The young woman GP said it was terrible news, that I had leukaemia. She had never had to tell a patient anything like this before and really didn't know what to do with herself. It ended up with me reassuring her that I would be okay."

Amanda paused, her head turning as her gaze followed the flight of a duck coming in to splash down noisily on the water in front of us. She was silent for moment then turned and looked directly into my eyes.

"It was like being struck by lightning. My mind stopped, all words and thinking ceased. I couldn't move, sat still and numbed. I had been taken into a different reality.

"As my mind started to work again, so the questions began to form. How long did I have? When would I die? What would it be like? The doctor couldn't give me any answers, saying I would need to see a consultant at the hospital to find out more and see what treatment was available.

"The waiting was unbearable. I tried to find out what it all meant, what was ahead of me. All I came up with were a few medical articles in the library which didn't give me anything I could really understand. They were all about the blood system, red and white corpuscles and platelets. Nothing about how I would feel or what it would be like.

"Eventually I was given an appointment at the hospital. Actually it wasn't a long wait but it felt like months. I spent hours being prodded and pushed and having unspeakably horrible things done to get a bone marrow sample. The doctors were very friendly and explained that leukaemia is cancer of the blood and bone marrow. They said the drugs would control it and in time I would be able to carry on as usual. All I would need to do was to turn up for appointments and take the drugs prescribed. Apart from that I should live life as normally as possible."

She told me all this in a matter of fact way, with no trace of anger about being treated in such an impersonal manner.

I felt angry on her behalf. "That's the medical profession. I've often heard it said that doctors are taught to see patients as a set of bodily organs that need putting right, rather than as real people struggling to live as best they can."

"Well, yes. And the difficulty for me was that I did not feel normal. Having a life threatening illness with death never far away is not conducive to normality. In truth it focuses the mind wonderfully. But no one could tell me what I could do apart from just be ill. There was no information about how to live with such terrible knowledge. I asked about counselling and was told, 'only when you are terminally ill, near the end.' It was a hellish time."

Just hearing her talk about it was certainly making my mind focus. What would it mean for me to live with someone with such a life sentence? How long would it last? What would it be like? Somehow I had avoided asking myself these questions. It didn't seem right to ask her either. And would it be any easier if I knew what was to come? Sometimes it's best not to know too much. Perhaps I could trust that my natural sensitivity along with what I had learned would be enough to see me through. I had said I wanted a journey into the unknown and that's what I had been given. Now I just had to get on with it.

I shivered, feeling cool. I don't know how long we had sat there, but the sun had moved over and we were in the shade.

"How about tea and cakes at the Jericho cafe? We need something sweet after all that intensity. Then we could go and see a film, take the focus off ourselves for a while."

7

Two days later we came back to the subject of her illness. This time we were in the car on our way to a clown meeting in London. It was a grey wet morning as we left Oxford, and I asked her what happened after she was over the initial shock of her diagnosis.

"My flatmate Jane had been bringing in loads of books and magazines that she thought might be helpful and I came across an article about the Bristol Cancer Help Centre which seemed to have a different approach. They said that cancer affects everything about us, not just isolated bits of our bodies. It was such a relief to find someone saying what I instinctively knew to be true. It went on to say that instead of being passive patients we could take charge of our lives and our treatment and completely change the experience of illness. I found that an amazing idea and sent for their brochure. When I got it I read that cancer care requires not only medical treatment but also care for the mind, the spirit, the emotions, the heart and the soul. Those words really spoke to me deeply and I decided to go for a visit."

"Extraordinary! What a revelation."

"It was more than that. I met several different advisers who explained to me that there was so much I could be doing to help myself while the doctors were doing their work. One of them told me I should try out homeopathy and acupuncture which could positively affect my general physical and emotional health. A dietician explained how diet has a major effect on our health and suggested I cut back on fried foods, sugar and fats. A counsellor recommended seeing a psychotherapist to work on all the emotional issues that were coming up. Someone else suggested taking up meditation and thinking about my spiritual life. I began to realise that instead of seeing myself as a helpless victim of a torturous illness I could choose to take charge of things. There was a whole world of new experiences to explore and my illness could become an enriching journey through life."

"That was a big turning point in your thinking."

"Yes, I left there with a new sense of hope and my head full of ideas. I realised it was time for me to grow up and take responsibility for my life. I would have to work out what I really wanted to do and how I wanted to live. I would make up for having a short life by living it to the full, whatever that might mean. I was not going to let my life pass in an unconscious blur."

"I sort of understand that," I said. "I only began to think about my life more consciously when things were going badly wrong with my family at home. I felt under so much stress that I just had to get away and find some peace and help. My explorations were about my emotions and spiritual life. I never thought of acupuncture and homeopathy as something for me."

"That's often the way it works. People carry on as they always have until something goes wrong, they get ill, have an accident, or have a family breakup. It's the shock that seems to wake them up to wonder about the meaning of their lives."

"Going back to the Cancer Centre, what happened afterwards?"

"Well, then I understood the sort of things I had to do, and I knew my time was limited. My life was not to be an endless opportunity and I really might die in a few years. The first thing I did was to go to see a homeopath. That was quite an experience. She asked about my life in great detail, not just my physical symptoms. She wanted to know all sorts of things about my character, my habits and how I was living, saying that all of these affect my health. That in itself was a revelation, realising how different it was from a visit to my doctor. Then I had these tiny pills to take. To my surprise they really had an effect on how I felt. I guess I was lucky to find such a wise healer who also became my teacher, and I've been seeing her ever since.

"Then I began to look for a psychotherapist. It took quite a time to find one I felt good about, and I have gone on seeing him regularly ever since. Rob really saved my life. He helped me through all the difficult times, sorting out my thinking and feelings. He was always there when I needed him, and even when I was in the isolation ward for all that time we had phone sessions every week.

"But I still had to deal with the medical profession, see the doctors. In some ways I am lucky as there is something special about oncologists. In general I find they are sensitive and respectful and I can really talk about my situation. I asked my consultant to be honest with me about how things were going as I wanted to know as much as possible, even though it could be difficult at times. I wanted to have all the information so I could be in charge of my treatment and make my own choices."

"And what about your every day life? Work and things? Did that change?"

"Completely. I went to work for Christian Aid, went to India, discovered a whole new world for myself. My spiritual life became much more important and for a time I lived in the ashram of an Indian guru known as Amma. I thought I would stay there for good but my health got worse and I couldn't get the treatment I needed, so I had to come back to England and the National Health Service. Then I found this job in Devon, discovered Sacred Clowning and began to think about serious writing."

"Oh, yes. You changed your whole life."

"In some sense everything has changed while in other ways it's all the same. I still have the illness, still take the drugs, but on the mental, emotional and spiritual levels I feel healed. I wake up every day with a sense of wonder and feel it's a gift to be alive. I am doing the best I can with what I've been given, and that's the most important thing anyone can do."

"One other thing," she added. "Just don't ever call me brave, or tell me I am courageous in the face of such difficulties. I can't stand that. This is not bravery, I'm just living the best way I can."

She was so open about all her experiences. I found it intensely moving to be given such an intimate account of her life. I was in awe of the way she had moved through it and grown in awareness, and it put my own life difficulties into a new perspective. It made me think more about how I had lived. Staying in my old marriage, I had let things drift. At least I was out of that, and was starting a new journey with Amanda.

8

July turned into August and we enjoyed getting closer. We went for more walks by the river and out in the countryside, explored the old town, met friends and tried to plan how we would live together. We became more intimate. We were physically attracted to each other and began a delightful journey into exploring each other's bodies.

In September we moved into a little terraced cottage in East Oxford, pooling our possessions, a few of mine from my old home and Amanda's from the warehouse where they had been stored. The house was near the Cowley Road, a lively area full of people of all nationalities and independent shops of every sort. Not far away were the university buildings in the centre of the city, built of warm yellow sandstone, standing on cobbled streets and little back lanes. Oxford is a city humming with life, with music, theatres, cinemas and green parks beside the river. It's a city for cycling and we loved being out on our bikes. We were so happy to be living there, and our joy was enhanced by the long hot summer.

We took our time to unpack and settle in, wanting to fully experience our coming together, becoming partners, discovering each others habits and ways of thinking and feeling. We made the house attractive, went shopping for bedding, a chest of drawers and a vacuum cleaner. Life was easy except that at times Amanda felt over-tired and needed to rest.

We went for walks in the moonlight and talked till late at night, diving deep into our new found intimacy. We shared our fears and worries about being in this relationship. I was still surprised at myself getting involved with someone so soon after leaving my marriage, and Amanda worried about how her health might affect things as time went on. I found it a delight to be with her. I had not had such an experience of openness and intimacy with a woman in my whole life, nor had I found such an enjoyable and relaxed way to live from day to day.

Friends came to see us. The clowns told me how different this all felt from the day they came to visit me at my old house.

We had our differences. We both enjoyed cooking, but had quite different styles. She was very careful about her diet, liked freshly steamed vegetables and rice, not much meat, little salt and no fried food. I was more of a traditional English cook, liking my eggs and bacon, toast and coffee. It took me time to realise she was a more thoughtful cook than me, and I began to appreciate the delicacies she created.

She didn't like the smell of my occasional cigarette so I agreed not to smoke in the house. I created a little den at the bottom of the back garden where I would go for a cigarette, and generally find a sense of peace sitting there amongst the shrubs. Nature has a calming touch and sometimes being in that place of peace and beauty was exactly what I needed.

Although she had passed her driving test she had no confidence in her ability to drive. I encouraged her, took her out for practice so she could have the freedom to go off on her own when she wanted.

One day I had a phone call from my old college inviting me to do some part time teaching, a counselling class and some staff development work with other teachers. I knew I would enjoy these and was glad to have the opportunity to earn some money.

"I want to find a job too," said Amanda, "both for the money and for the social contact that it would bring. I don't like being on benefits and struggling with the social pressure to 'fight your illness and work for your living'. But, I'm afraid I am unemployable. My health goes up and down so much and I can't imagine who would want to employ me."

She did apply for several part time jobs but no-one offered her a post. Though she understood the reasons she was angry at the prejudice she felt lay behind the rejections.

Meanwhile in our daily life together it was not all easy going. Sometimes she would snap at me for no apparent reason, and I would feel hurt and angry.

"One of the many side effects of my drugs is that they cause a sort of early menopause, and that brings more symptoms such as unpredictable mood swings. Sometimes I simply feel irritable, and it is nothing to do with you. You just happen to be the person in the firing line!"

It was hard to remember this all the time. I would find myself reacting strongly to some comment she made, feeling angry that she had misunderstood me. I still took it all personally, felt she was blaming me as if I had done something wrong. That was when I would head off down the garden for a smoke, to nurse my wounded feelings. Then, later in the day, we would come together and unravel the crazy stories we had been creating in our minds, and resolve to try to be more aware of what was going on between us.

We enjoyed living in Oxford with its alternative community and rich variety of things to do. We went to Chi Gung classes in a hall nearby and then on to the Magic Cafe with others from the class to enjoy quiche and salad, and talk of this and that. We browsed the shelves of the Inner Bookshop, looking for wisdom and entertainment.

Amanda bought me a copy of The Shaman's Way by Arnold Mindell. In it he expresses ideas about the interconnectedness of every facet of life. He shows the links between our feelings, our night time dreams, our physical symptoms, things that happen to us and events in the world at large. He offers an understanding of life that includes modern psychology, quantum physics, human intuition and the study of shamanism. I was fascinated and we talked about going to his workshops later in the year.

She also gave me a book about Amma, the guru she had followed when she was in India, explaining that she was considered to be a living saint in her own land. I read how Amma had grown up as a poor peasant child who had wanted to follow in the path of Krishna, and had gone on to start her own ashram and eventually to run huge charities doing good works for the poor of India. Amanda told me that now, every year, Amma comes to London for a three-day ceremony and people come in thousands to see her and receive darshan, a blessing, from her in the form of a big enveloping embrace.

Amma was due to come to England soon and Amanda suggested we go to the ceremonies at Battersea town hall. We went to stay with a friend who lived near the hall and walked over every day. I had never been in such a gathering and felt very stimulated by the vibrancy, colour and movement of all the people there from all over the world. I loved sitting with everyone on the floor, chanting Bhajans, listening to Amma's talk, the candlelight, the music. I felt I could surrender to a spiritual presence here, knowing that life is much more than I could understand.

We sat in the queue of people waiting our turn to receive darshan, while there was music and singing all around. We went up together to ask for her blessing on our lives and relationship. Amma received us and enfolded us together in her arms, whispering blessings in our ears. I felt a flow of love and knew we would be helped.

I was very taken by that event. It was the first time I had been to a Hindu ceremony with so much life, activity and music, and the first time I had met a living holy person. What a contrast to the formal sedate rituals of the Christian church.

With so much going on in our lives, so many new experiences and things to think about I had almost forgotten about Amanda's illness, so it was a shock when, a few days later, she said she needed to talk about her health. We were sitting in the kitchen after breakfast, and she said:

"I have a new lump."

Alarm and fear instantly ran through my body, gripping my heart and guts.

"I'm afraid it's serious and tells me I could be getting worse. I'm frightened. It brings up all my fears and worries. My leukaemia could be turning from chronic to acute. I could be going to die soon."

I tried to calm myself, not to go into panic. I had to search for words. "Oh no. That's awful, terrible. Are there any other signs?"

"Yes, look. It's here, and I feel weak and sick."

I looked at and felt the swelling which seemed quite small and couldn't help wondering if a new lump was a sure sign of such a change. How I wished I had more medical knowledge.

"I'm afraid of dying."

Tears sprang to her eyes, and to mine.

"This fear is so overwhelming. It's been with me for years. It's even more poignant now when I have so much to live for: our relationship, the clowning, my writing and singing. I don't want to die, I want to live."

We sat, looking into each others eyes, both feeling overwhelmed.

There was little more we could do except to arrange to see the consultant as soon as possible. It took a few days to get an appointment, days of anxiety and worry with little to alleviate it.

We drove to St Thomas' hospital and I sat in the windowless waiting room with its bare yellow walls. Leafing through old magazines I held back my fear while she went for blood tests, then to see the registrar and then finally to see the consultant.

When she came out she sat to tell me what he had said, and it all came out in a rush.

"He didn't say much about the new lump, but the results of my blood tests are not good. I have too many white blood cells and not enough red ones. However they are fairly stable which tells me that nothing is changing at the moment and I am not in such danger. That's good, but I want to get the blood counts up. He says the medication may do that."

So much information in one breath. It took me a moment to work out what she had said, that she was not in danger.

"Does that mean it is not turning acute?"

"Yes, that's what I said, but there is still a lot to be worried about."

"But I thought …" I stopped. I had spent the whole morning in fear and worry about the diagnosis and that had left me feeling sick inside. I wanted to say how pleased I was that she was not worse, but I still had this heavy sick feeling in my guts. It was if she had forgotten all that worrying, had already moved on to deal with the new reality.

"I'm not sure about the medication," she went on, "I have just as much trust in acupuncture and homeopathy. I must make appointments as soon as I can."

"OK, but let's go and have a cup of coffee first. I'm desperate for something to perk me up."

In the cafe I reminded her of how worried we had been all last week and told her of my fears while waiting for her, and how that had left me feeling sick.

"I thought you were rather quiet. I understand now. I'm sorry that happened."

That night in my room I took out my journal to write about the day. At the end I wrote: I am so confused. I find it hard to believe in the reality of her illness although it is so clearly real, perhaps because there is nothing to actually see. I have no experience that comes anywhere near it. I can empathise, try to come close to her feelings, but it is too enormous. The hardest is if I begin to imagine the future and how her illness might develop. At those times I don't know if I am crying for her suffering or my loss. In the end it seems we are on a journey together into the unknown, living and exploring, finding our way through our lives that may bring anything from joy, love, pain, misery and despair mixed with hope and wonder. I feel this is a gift to me, a rare experience of life that is bringing me closer to deeper truths.

9

In October we went on a four-day seminar in Process Work run by Arny Mindell. It was a large, energetic affair involving movement, dance, talk, bodywork, shamanism and more. He is a brilliant, creative and relaxed facilitator. I felt my mind being opened and expanded in quite unfamiliar ways. At one stage he led us all into a kind of shamanic dream journey which took me deep into my unconscious. Near the end of it I seemed to be looking into a river of deep flowing water. At that moment Arny said, "What you see now is who you are." I was looking at a river and I understood the message to be "I am River." I felt at once that this was true, that it was a reflection of my true nature. I thought to myself that River was my real name, the one that expressed the truth of my being. My given name, Nick, seemed nothing more than a label that had been attached to me, a bit like Paddington Bear.

Over the following days I explored the imagery of the name to see where it fitted. Yes, like a river I can be fast and wild, slow and deep, shallow and noisy. My life does make sudden changes of direction, goes over waterfalls, has rocky periods, and all the time it is running out towards the ocean. Every river is a unique mix of moving water and fixed banks, of fish and plant life and can never be fully known.

Humans too are unique and can never be fully known. I was deeply touched by the name, found it a helpful image in understanding my life. I thought about using it in public but didn't feel ready for it. It was as if the name was something I could aspire to in the future, not a recognition of something I had already become.

Amanda liked the name. We thought it could also be a metaphor for our lives together, the two of us paddling down an uncharted river in a canoe, never knowing what might be round the next corner. We knew we were in a mountainous country and might meet rapids and waterfalls at any time, but there could be pools of deep calm water where we could rest and be at peace. We decided to study Process Work more seriously, and planned to go to more training events.

She introduced me to the Tao Te Ching, an ancient book of Chinese philosophy. There was something about the opening words that felt deeply significant: 'The Tao that can be told is not the eternal Tao. The name that can be named is not the eternal name.' I sat to meditate on them and often returned to contemplate other chapters of the book.

She showed me how to 'throw the I Ching'. Based on the Book of Changes, it's an ancient Chinese system used to bring deeper understanding of whatever situation we find ourselves in. It also offers insights in to what are the most helpful ways to move forward at the present time.

In November we had another weekend with Lex and the other clowns. Being together with them brought delight and a sense of fun. This time there was a lot of improvised singing. I loved hearing Amanda, Val and Susan improvising together, three beautiful voices entwining in a glory of harmonies. Later I joined a larger group singing together and enjoyed myself, but sensed I was not appreciated. "Perhaps you could sing more softly," suggested Susan. "When you sing you should always be able to hear what everyone else is doing, that way you stay in touch with them rather than overpowering them."

It took me a minute to take in what she was saying. I hadn't realised I actually needed to listen to the other singers in order to harmonise. How naïve of me. Then I began to wonder about other situations I might not be listening. I also wondered about the sort of things I might be saying without realising it.

Amanda said. "Use your voice to express what is inside you. Try singing from your heart. Open your mouth and let your voice sing what your heart feels. Give no thought to what is right or wrong, good or bad, just let the sounds come." This was all new, quite different from my school day singing. I tried to do as she suggested but found it hard. The sounds I made were more of a low groaning wailing sound, slurring from one note to another. Maybe that was all my heart had to say just then.

Thinking about it, living with Amanda and going to the psychology workshops and the clowning were certainly making me have a fresh look at myself.

A week later I had my first ever acupuncture treatment to work on pains I had been feeling in my stomach. The treatment was so strange, sticking tiny pins into different parts of my body and I couldn't believe it would do anything.

That evening I began to feel dizzy and then almost high. I fell asleep and woke feeling delirious. Amanda stayed with me and after a while I came down and then felt quite clear headed and well balanced. That feeling stayed with me over the coming days, the pains in my stomach disappeared, and more than that I found I had lost any desire for a cigarette, alcohol or coffee.

I remembered the dream I'd had in the summer when I was promised transformation if I chose to make a life with Amanda. With everything I had gone through in the last three months I felt I was on a course of major change and growth.

But Amanda was finding she had less energy and was feeling weak. She spent more time lying in bed, watching television and hadn't been doing any writing.

"I don't feel well, can't sleep because of restless legs," she said. "I feel depressed and I'm worried and afraid because all my symptoms and feelings go on and on and there's just no ending. I am completely losing my body shape and my clothes don't fit me properly, and it's impossible to find anything at all fashionable to wear. I have no income and we are living on your earnings and savings. I don't feel well enough to work and I'm afraid I may never feel strong enough to work again. Everything depresses me these days."

"What do you feel now about the Buddhist idea of surrendering to what is, accepting that this is the reality we are in? They say that wanting it to be different is what causes us problems?"

"It's a wonderful concept but hard to put into practice, particularly when 'what is' is so unpleasant and 'what might be' is so attractive. We are so accustomed to having a good life, it's hard to accept one that is not so good. And what does it mean in my daily life? What do I do with myself every day?

And what does it suggest I do about money? I am only getting unemployment benefit and you know how little that is. We are struggling and I'm wondering if I should apply for disability benefit."

We wondered how we might work together and perhaps make some money running clowning workshops and performances.

"But how can I commit myself if I don't know if I will be well enough to do them?"

"Difficult. I don't see how we could plan something together, knowing that I might have to do it alone?"

We began to wonder about getting a small clowning group together, just a few people who would be interested in starting a clown business. With more people it might be easier to manage Amanda's unpredictable health.

So we rang our friends Val, Phil and Carola and suggested we get together to talk about the idea. A week later we met for an afternoon to discuss the possibilities. They were enthusiastic and we agreed to start meeting regularly and to organise ourselves as a proper clown group that would put on performances and run workshops. We decided to call ourselves Fools Gold.

10

Christmas came and went. There were a few parties and we visited members of each other's families.

In January Amanda had one of her regular appointments at St Thomas' hospital to see the Professor, the one she liked and respected, who would tell it like it is. We drove up and I waited as she went through the long drawn-out process of blood tests, seeing the registrar and then the Professor. I sat in the familiar yellow waiting room leafing through magazines and by the time she was done I was feeling drained and sleepy.

She looked pale and tense as she sat down. "He told me its not good news. Things are getting worse and they are wondering which would be the best way to deal with it. There are no easy options."

I forced myself to wake up, to give attention to what she was saying. "What does that mean?"

"I have to make choices about my treatment. I could go for another bone marrow transplant, but I know what that's like and don't want to go through it all again." Another pause. "I could try the drug interferon but they say it can have awful side effects. Otherwise I can carry on as I am, and slowly go downhill. The truth is none of these appeals or sounds very hopeful."

But that wasn't all.

"This is what the professor said to me: *I am afraid it's clear that your illness is progressing and will lead at some time to your death.*"

"Oh, I see. How much longer do you think I have?"

"*I can't say exactly, but you should be thinking in terms of months rather than years.*"

Amanda paused.

Her words instantly struck home to my heart. My guts sank. Hope slipped away.

She looked into my eyes.

"Oh. I'm so sorry. That's awful to hear."

Nothing I could say would make any difference, but I knew that just being there and loving her was a help in itself. I needed to be there, to witness what she was going through.

We sat, silent. Our eyes said it all.

Somehow we got out of the waiting room and down to the cafe where we ordered cups of hot chocolate. Not just ordinary hot chocolate from a tin but real freshly made intense tasting rich dark hot chocolate. That helped to lift our spirits.

I don't remember the drive home. Somehow we held on and got through the journey and the days that followed. Gradually we found ourselves coming closer and more tender towards each other, taking pleasure in our sensuality together, lying in each others arms and making sweet love, with an ever more intimate connection that was both spiritual and physical.

But my mind kept slipping off into the future, imagining all the possible pain and suffering that was to come. Each time I brought myself back to the present moment, to simply being here.

The choice of treatment did not go away. A few weeks later we went again to the hospital for more tests and talk. They said she needed to make the decision about what treatment to opt for.

We talked and held each other. I cried.

"These tears just keep coming and I can't control them".

"Why would you want to control them? You are just letting out your real feelings. You know sometimes you have to simply surrender to what life brings. That's not giving up. That's accepting that this is the way your life is going, the way your soul needs to go."

"But I'm so unsure of myself. Can I really deal with all this? Will I be able to cope with things as you get more ill?"

"Actually I'm glad you're telling me what you are afraid of. It reminds me that you too are human, have lots of self doubt."

"But my mind goes round and round. What if it goes on for years? What if the drugs cause a personality change and you start behaving weirdly? What if I run out of money and we can't afford to stay here? I want to be here with you and for you, but life is too mysterious, and I don't want to make promises that later I can't keep."

"It's OK. Let's just accept that these are fantasies, they are not real. Let's stay with reality. And if things do change we will find our way through."

It was a relief to be honest about what was in my mind, even though part of me thought I should keep my fears secret, for fear that these 'bad' thoughts would only make things worse. I guess that came from the way I was brought up, to only show the 'nice' parts of my character. But honesty and openness were going to be the best ways for us to get through it all. I felt we were like two children on a journey through a huge forest where there were no paths. We just had to go on hand in hand and hope for the best. We talked and we cried. I was getting used to having a lump in my throat, a sniffy nose and tears in my eyes.

I tried not to lay all the weight of my difficult thoughts and feelings on Amanda. I talked to my friends about my feelings. David calmly accepted that this was just how my life was at the time. Val and Carola were warm and understanding. Acupuncture helped me too, working like magic to add to my inner sense of balance.

I had started seeing a new psychotherapist. Jean Claude was one of the Process Work teachers and I found him open hearted and easy to talk with. He listened to me and validated my feelings and responses. He helped me find new perspectives, to step back a little from my emotional swamp, to see that this was all part of being human. It would be inhuman of me to try to suppress it all. I liked his approach, but I still struggled. It ran so counter to all of my upbringing and culture to let other people see what was really going on deep inside.

I found support too through my meditation practice. I was meditating most mornings, sitting quietly on a cushion in the front room, sometimes with a candle and Nag Champa incense. It helped me to manage my mind better, so I didn't get lost in the sad stories about the future running through my head, and repeating over and over again. Meditation interrupted all that and left me feeling calm and peaceful.

Spring came and turned out to be an easier time with many things to do, and plenty of space within to do them slowly. We had a short holiday in Majorca staying with a friend, then a Process Workshop in Leeds and visits with friends. We went to clown gatherings, relaxing and playing together, and prepared for more public performances in the future. But there were the regular visits to hospital that always reminded me of the realities we were facing.

Money was becoming a problem and the rent was high. It's true we spent a lot on our various activities but they were important for both of us and we didn't want to cut back on them. My teaching work at the college helped but was not enough. I tried the usual ways to find a means to make money. I read the job adverts in the newspaper but found nothing I was drawn to. I thought over the various jobs I had done over the years but there was nothing that I wanted to go back to. We began to realise we would have to find a cheaper place to live, perhaps not in Oxford.

None the less, I felt very alive, more richly so than ever before. I wrote in my journal:

> *I feel human, loving, loved*
> *Weak and vulnerable, strong and able*
> *Full of doubt and uncertainty*
> *Hopeful and fearful*
> *Aware and awake.*

11

I wrote more in my journal: Is it enough to just be living as we are, going from day to day without any particular direction? Am I just drifting through my life? Shouldn't I take charge of it? I have no sense of ambition, no desire to develop my career. It's the difference between Being and Doing. I am someone who is often content to simply Be, have no need to Do anything. And that is not the way our society works. We are all expected to want to do things, to achieve something worthwhile.

There are times when I think I want to achieve, would like to find something I could really put my energy into, perhaps play a fuller part in society and the world. But I don't know how I would do that. I need to feel inspired, attracted to some occupation. And that, I think, will come somehow from inside. Too often in the past I have taken up some interest only for it to fade after a few months. I don't want to do that again. There seems to be some deeper drive in me, something unconscious, that decides how my life will develop. It's not up to my thinking mind to find a new direction. I believe it will become clear if I remain open-minded and receptive, perhaps through a dream, an intuition or some chance meeting with someone. But then I get impatient, want to know now, not sometime in the future.

I also wrote: I think about life a lot these days. I wonder how much the love I feel for Amanda is intensified by her illness. If she did not have it, if our lives felt more open ended, would I feel so strongly about her? Would we even have started to live together?

Books were important to me and I was reading a lot. I had Ken Wilber's book Grace and Grit about his experience of living with his wife who was diagnosed with cancer. I liked what he says about the Inner Witness, 'one's innate capacity to simply witness phenomena.' You don't always have to have a response to what happens, you can just observe it. At first I had thought it was unfeeling but actually it just means that it is sometimes okay for me to be with Amanda when she's suffering, and not go through any mental or emotional reaction. I can simply be there with her.

The book made me think about how widely she had been exploring ways to deal with her illness. Naturally she wanted to be free of pain, but she saw that the whole process went far beyond the purely physical aspects of life. Healing for her was more than just getting back to the state of physical health she was in before it all started. It meant growing into a place of fullness in heart, mind and spirit. So clowning and spirituality were as important as acupuncture and homeopathy. I had never thought in such broad ways, having generally left my health either to luck or the medical profession.

Steven Levine's book Who Dies? was beside my bed. It offered me fresh insights into what it means to be fully alive, and a new way of understanding what it means to die, and to die consciously. I came back to this book many times and always found it helpful.

Around that time we went on a reiki training course. We learned to sit beside the other person with our hands on their body so that natural healing energy could pass through you to them. I was sceptical about the explanations we were given, but found that sitting still with my hands on the 'patient' was both powerful and calming. It seemed to bring about a subtle connection between the giver and the receiver. After that Amanda and I often gave each other reiki, and that gave me a sense that there was something I could do that would help her healing, as well as being something I could receive from her. Sometimes our friends Val and Syd came round and we all gave her reiki at the same time.

Amanda arranged for her medical treatment to be transferred to the John Radcliffe hospital in Oxford to be nearer to home. For her appointment in March I suggested I come in to see the consultant with her as a support. She had always seen her doctors alone in the past, but agreed that now it might be a good idea. This was a significant change, an opening to what she had always kept private. I felt more deeply trusted and the consultation gave me a greater insight to her condition and what she was living through. He suggested a new drug that had just come on the market which he thought would be helpful but could have difficult side effects. He left it up to her to decide whether she wanted to try it or not.

We talked about this question. I couldn't find a way to help her make this choice. It felt like gambling. How could one decide which way to go when even the doctor prescribing the drug did not know what it would do?

We talked about the problem of having so many different sorts of treatment available and how one makes choices, not just about medical drugs but the whole range of alternative therapies too. It was impossible to get an overview of how they would all interact. And it is all skewed by the medical profession which believes that it is the only real player in the field. It is so huge and powerful with its huge impressive buildings, ranges of scientific equipment, specialists and vast budgets, and is very scathing of alternatives. How can the offerings of a homeopath in his shed compete with this? And yet we knew these other treatments have so much to offer.

She decided to see what other therapists had to say.

She went to see her homeopath and talked about her options. But there was no clear answer.

She went to see the well-known psychic healer Keith Casburn. He was helpful but he couldn't advise her which way to go either.

We talked more about her illness.

"How do you actually feel about it on a daily basis?" I ask. "With all this talk of treatments I'm losing touch with how you feel on this inside. How much of the time do you think about Leukaemia?"

"It's always with me, yet most of the time I'm not really aware of it. The worst times are at night when all the fears and worries rise up. That happens when I sleep alone, less so when we sleep together. But the fear can be overwhelming. I worry that the doctors might be right and I should try their latest drugs? Could I be leaving it too late and go past some point of no return to where nothing more can be done?"

12

In the morning we were having our breakfast of muesli and coffee by the window in our little kitchen, and we returned yet again to the unresolved question.

"It's still no clearer," she sighed. "They don't know what to do and I don't know what to do."

"There's still the acupuncture and homeopathy," I said hopefully.

"Oh yes, and all the personal and emotional stuff I do. But does it really help? Should I carry on with it all? I just don't know." She smiled. "Perhaps, I should give in to the inevitable, take the latest wonder drug, put up with the side effects and eat as much chocolate as I want!"

We laughed. Sometimes, with such imponderables upon us, humour was all we had to keep us going. It was a way for us to keep talking to each other and share our worries in a more light hearted way.

I reached out and took her hand. "Well, we are in this together. I feel just as lost and confused. I'm sorry I don't know how you make such a choice."

She drew back. "That doesn't help much! Everything is telling me I'm on a downward slope and I need you to be more encouraging, help lift me out of despair."

"It's difficult. I don't know what to say. I am here with you on this journey. Deep down I know this is what I need to be doing with my life and I know that there is a spiritual significance to our living together and experiencing life as it is." I started to do a little clowning improvisation about our situation, creating an image of the two of us sitting miserably side by side, then gradually sinking, slipping down onto the floor and curling up into a shrivelled ball of misery. It made us both laugh and brought some lightness and relief.

"Actually, I'm getting in a real muddle over it all," I said. "Whose life are we living? Sometimes it seems that my life has been put on hold. I am in this with you all the way, but it has taken over everything. I give so much time to thinking about you that I forget my own needs. Maybe that is why I feel so despairing. I feel overloaded with caring. I seem to spend my life driving you from appointment to appointment, sitting in waiting rooms and listening to your problems. I too have a life to live. I need to give some attention to myself, and would like some attention from you as well."

"Well, yes. I can see that. You do need to look after yourself. You should take more time out, go and do the things that you enjoy. As Lex would say, follow your passion".

"I need to find a balance between supporting you and meeting my own needs."

"Yes, I don't want you to become 'the carer' while I am the 'needy one'. I want us both to live our lives fully whatever comes. We have to each stay with our own truths. Only by doing that can we be in a real and authentic relationship."

I decided I would do that, take more time away from her, to just be myself.

I made an appointment to see Pam, my acupuncturist. That might help build my energy and lift me out of apathy and depression. Pam talked of how Amanda and I act as a counterbalance for each other so one can go into the extremes of feeling while the other holds us safely on the ground. I found that helpful, and a good reminder that we were both on this journey. In the drama of her serious illness I easily forgot that I too was profoundly affected, even though I was not threatened with physical death.

I was glad I still had my teaching work that took me away from home. I was running some staff development sessions which were both challenging and stimulating and my counselling class was going well. Several of the participants talked about changes and improvements in their lives that had come about as a result of the course. It was pleasing to feel I was playing a part in the world at large as well as in our private home life.

I decided I needed to get more exercise, so I joined the Oxford Town rowing club. I used to row when I was at school and particularly loved sculling. It only took me a couple of outings to regain my confidence and then I was free to paddle down the river. I loved the feeling of my muscles working purposefully together and delighted in the way the fine boat slipped through the water. It gave me time on my own and a chance to come closer to nature and the wild life on the river.

Amanda and I looked for more outside interests we could enjoy together. We joined a Process Work study group looking at Arny Mindell's book 'Sitting in the Fire'. The lively conversations we had took our minds off our problems to think about the bigger world issues of the time. The group helped us to see how our personal lives were not so different from the lives and problems of all peoples around the world. Working on our journey with leukaemia was just another aspect of the difficulties everyone faces, simply as a consequence of living in the world with other people. Knowing this made me feel more confident about talking openly to others about our sometimes difficult processes. I began to see that it could be helpful to others to see how we were dealing with our situation.

One day after breakfast I was feeling tired and sat reading a book in the sitting room when Amanda came down feeling lively and energetic. She wanted to talk about the last meeting we had been to, but I wanted to go on reading and didn't feel like getting into a conversation. I felt I ought to respond to her but just couldn't, and instead went off upstairs to my bedroom.

That afternoon she said, "This seems to be a pattern with us, we are like a see-saw, one is energetic and the other tired, and we seem to have lost our joint creativity. What is happening to us? Is our relationship somehow stifling us?"

She suggested we explore this using clowning and the Process Work techniques we had studied. That seemed a good idea and we started to act out our feelings. She began to dance her energy, while I slowly collapsed into a tired heap on the floor. We exaggerated these through movement and gestures. Gradually we found that we were moving apart, quite unconsciously. As this happened my energy picked up, until finally we were in separate rooms and I, too, was dancing with lots of energy. So there we were, both dancing, but in different rooms.

"This suggests we need to live a bit more separately," she said.

"Well, that's the way it looks. But how can we do that in such a small house?"

We realised that we both felt different when we were alone in the house. Just the knowledge that the other is there in another room changes things, though neither of us could define exactly how. We each needed our own separate spaces. Not being a couple who could do everything together, we needed to be able to be alone by ourselves and also to meet with friends without the other being there.

"I don't know how we'll manage in the future if my health gets worse and I become more dependent on you."

"Yes, that might be a problem, but let's not worry about it now. It's just another thing we will have to try to stay conscious about."

We talked more about moving house. Not only did we need to save money but now we also wanted a bigger place to live in. A trip round the estate agents confirmed we could not afford anywhere reasonable in Oxford, so we began to look for places further away.

I went to see Jean Claude. Sometimes we simply talked, trying to gain deeper awareness and understanding of what life is bringing me. At other times he encouraged me to go into the unknown parts of my mind, a bit like dreaming, but done awake and consciously. On this occasion I had an ache in my back and he asked me to put my attention there. As I began to focus on the ache I felt the pain grow and become almost unbearable until I was groaning and tears were running down my face. After a while this slowed and reduced, and I found myself coming into a sense of lightness and relief, as if I had released something, let go of some burden I did not need to hold on to any more. I left the session feeling restored and uplifted, knowing that somehow this related to my life with Amanda.

That good feeling stayed with me at home, and was particularly noticeable when Amanda was feeling irritable and I was able to stay on an even keel. Later she explained that it was the drugs that had made her feel awful and bad tempered and that my calm and positive presence had been helpful.

13

In June we went to see a house in Banbury, much bigger and cheaper. It was an old Victorian three-story building with five bedrooms and two reception rooms. Quite enough to give us each our own space. It was a long way from our friends and our social life, but we both liked it, so we paid the deposit with the intention of moving in September.

In July we had a five-day Process workshop to go to. That was to be followed by several days on a clowning trip to Germany to meet some German clown students there and put on a joint performance. I felt excited about it all. I had almost forgotten about Amanda's illness and just assumed she would be okay. But a hospital check-up showed her blood count was even lower than before, which meant her Leukaemia was progressing.

"I don't know if I will be up to so much activity," she said. "Maybe I should stay here and you go off on your own."

I knew I ought to feel sorry for her, but actually I felt angry and frustrated. So much was going on that I wanted to do, and I wanted her to come and do it too. I was like a small child who wants to blame mummy for spoiling his plans.

At the same time I had that sinking feeling in my guts. I felt the time was drawing closer. It was as if we were living near the entrance to a long dark tunnel, but this one had no light at the end. We could be forced to go down it at any time.

"I am so fed up with always being ill," said Amanda. "I feel I am always being the damp rag at the party, the one who has to leave early. I can cope with the physical pain of it all, but it's the weakness and vulnerability that I hate most and the feeling of being sentenced to a lifetime of illness. I don't believe that any of the treatments available will help much." She was silent for a moment. "On top of that, I know I'm going to die sometime soon and I feel cheated that there is so much I will not be able to do. I feel cheated that you will live on and I will never see you as you grow old."

I didn't know what to say. I had to accept she was probably right and I would live on, without her. Tears filled my eyes, a swelling sensation blocked my throat.

"Look at me. I've got water retention in my legs and face, I feel so weak that even going upstairs is an effort. I feel as if my whole body is rearranging itself on the inside and has become unfamiliar. It's very frightening."

There followed difficult days when she went through rapid changes of mood and sudden emotional outbursts.

I felt confused and rejected when I seemed to be the target of all these feelings, but I was slowly learning to see that her explosions were not about me but were expressions of what was happening inside her.

I was becoming more aware of how she was feeling at different times and of what she might need. If she was in despair I understood that she might want to be held or just to know that I was there, or she might want to talk or just be on her own. I no longer tried to offer comforting answers. Sometimes I sat and admitted that things were unbearable and we cried together; at other times it seemed helpful to use humour to lighten the feelings.

And I got less pulled into Amanda's emotional state. There were times when she was struggling and in pain and I stayed feeling positive, not being drawn into her despair. She said that this was good for her. If she was depressed the last thing she wanted was for me to get depressed too.

I felt that being with her was my real work, was the most valuable thing I could be doing with my life. It took most of my attention and energy. I lived for the day, without much thought for the future. I had come to accept that this was my life and that there were certain things I could not change.

And I was more honest about my feelings. I no longer replied 'I'm doing fine' when someone asked. I told them how I was really feeling at that moment.

And then, unexpectedly, and for no apparent reason, her health improved. She felt better, more alive and energetic, wanted to go out and be in the world more. It felt as if the sun had come out. I enjoyed her company so much. And later we could climb into bed, cuddle and be warm and loving together. We were filled with joy and hope. Perhaps the doctors and their statistics really were wrong and her life would not be shortened as they predicted. We never did find out why that change happened, the doctors and therapists just put it down to the mysteries of the human body.

It meant she felt she could manage the Process workshop as long as we took care not to over do it. She thought she could probably cope with the trip to Germany, though perhaps not take part in all the activities, and that is what we did.

14

After a wonderful summer we moved to the house in Banbury.

Even though we arrived in a rainstorm and unloaded in the wet, the house was welcoming and we were full of hope and delight in this new beginning. It was a time of fresh opportunities, an opening out into the world.

It was not long before visitors arrived, some to stay a night or two. There were friends, family and clowns, and the house was filled with talking, singing and clowning. I told everyone they had to look after themselves, to bring and prepare food and do the clearing up afterwards as well as do their share of the laundry and cleaning. Everyone was fine with that and it worked well. I did have occasional thoughts that I should be a better host but actually I found I could relax quite easily while others were working in the kitchen.

Amanda was happy enjoying the company and closeness of her friends, and going off to her room when she needed to rest. Another good thing was discovering that Brenda, an old friend of hers, lived nearby and they met up every now and then.

Banbury itself is a small market town, nothing like Oxford,

with little to interest me apart from the old Banbury Cross. Some days I went out to explore the local countryside, but even that was uninspiring. It's flat and dull, quite tame with endless farm fields and trimmed hedges, but I enjoyed long walks on my own and did find one little place that the farmers had not touched. There was a little spring in an overgrown corner of a field and there I stopped to enjoy the flowers and birds and reflect on the unexpected twists and turns of the life I was living.

Amanda wanted to make new curtains for the huge bay windows in our sitting room and bedroom, and took us to London, to Brixton cloth market, to look for beautiful materials. Back home she took out her scissors and sewing machine and set to work with me as her assistant. The sitting room curtains were to be made of two layers of soft pink and green, while the bedroom curtains had a layer of white transparent netting with golden moons and stars over a thick deep blue material. We worked on these together when she had the energy.

She was also meeting up regularly with Didier and Lex to make plans for a book about clowning, and then taking her notes up to her office on the top floor to write it up. This was important creative work for her, and writing was one of the main pleasures of her life. Meanwhile I signed up for a photography class at the local college, enjoying developing and printing in the dark room and also an art class to open my eyes to really see what was in front of me. I found a flamenco dance class to go to in the evenings and that lifted my spirits. I loved the vibrant aliveness and strong presences, the powerful male and female energies meeting in dramatic movement.

Part Two

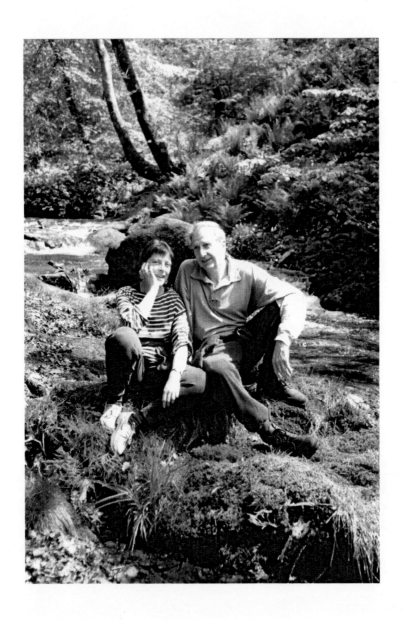

15

It's November. The days are shorter and it's wet and cold. Amanda is in pain and feeling sick. As the day goes on the pain gets worse. I sit with her, offer reiki along with touch and comfort. I encourage her to let out the pain, to cry and shout as much as she needs.

I cry and shout too, to let out this mixture of sadness and anger that is filling my body and heart.

She gets through the night but in the morning the pain is worse. The doctor comes but doesn't seem to know what to do. She has intense pain in her groin, can't walk or move about. She feels desperate, abandoned, confused, worthless, angry, afraid and hopelessly dependent on others. All the unanswered questions. How long? What if? Why now?

I drive her to hospital and they diagnose blood seeping into the muscles of her groin as the cause of the pain. They give her stronger painkillers, tell her to rest and that it should ease with time. We are free to go home.

It's agony for her and we are both in tears. The days seem endless. What can you do to pass the time in pain?

"I try to meditate and be with it," she says, "but there are times when I just want to veg out, to lose consciousness." She watches endless TV just to take her mind off it all.

It's different for me. I have so much to do apart from just being with her. I am responsible for our physical lives, I go shopping, prepare food, carry meals up to her bed, take plates down afterwards, and wash up. I tidy the house, make the beds, do the laundry, help her to the loo and bathroom and do mundane things like paying bills.

As the days turn into weeks I realise it's getting too much for me and I need some help. But I don't know how to get help, don't even know how to ask for it. A part of me says I don't really need it, that I can manage if I really try. Another part of me just wants to go off out somewhere, hang out with friends, have a beer and relax without any worries.

Amanda says she would like to do that too. But she is in too much pain and has no escape. She wants to have someone with her most of the time. "I like having friends to visit, but they don't really understand how it is for me. I feel so weak and vulnerable and feel safer when you are here. They don't understand my need for autonomy the way you do. Teresa is a good friend but when she was here and you were out she just took control of everything, and I felt completely disempowered. I hate it when that happens. Being in charge of my life is the most important thing for me."

But I can't be there all the time, I need to have breaks for my own sake. When friends come to visit I grab the opportunity to get out and do my own thing, even if it's just going for a walk and taking some photographs. My Monday evening flamenco class cheers me every time.

And when I do get time alone I find myself wondering more and more about our lives together. I keep asking myself about the meaning of pain. Why does she have to hurt so much? What purpose does it serve? This intense pain that wipes out all her ability to think and feel normally. Sometimes it feels like a deliberate torture, a cat playing with the mouse before the final crunch.

Then, when I am feeling more open minded, I think of the whole thing as a process of change, where she is being hammered into a new shape on some gigantic anvil in the heat of the forge of illness. Something greater is being created inside her. And it seems this cannot be done without incurring immense pain.

But at the same time the illness is destroying her, so she may not live to express this greatness. Not in this lifetime. Is there another?

And I ask what her pain means to me. It affects me deeply, I'm not just a casual observer. It's a drain on my energy, but is it something more? I begin to think that pain has no meaning in itself, but perhaps there is significance in how we respond to it? I know it influences the way I relate to Amanda. Without it our lives would have been quite different and I would not have grown as I have. I don't have her physical pain but I do struggle with my mind and feelings. Sometimes I feel that all my tears and grief are dissolving the hard insensitive parts of me. Perhaps through this suffering I too am becoming greater.

And I wonder about love. What is it that keeps me here, binds me to her? How do I know I love her? What are the inner feelings and sensations that tell me this is love? When I think about it, I am not aware of feeling anything most of the time. Of course there are peak occasions when things are either so joyful I am full of warmth or so desperate I am full of sadness. But perhaps love is not a constant, not a single feeling, its more the rise and fall, the flow of feelings. A river of love. It's what my heart demands and it brings its own fulfilment. Without that I am empty and without purpose.

Meanwhile outside in the everyday world nothing is different. The shops are busy, pubs are full and people carry on their normal lives, all unaware of the drama going on behind our front door. I think how often I have been too busy with my own life to listen and give attention to people in pain. How many other people are in pain behind their own front doors? How many people are caring for sick mothers, fathers, partners, children and more? I get a wider perspective on this world of caring, one that I had not known before.

After three weeks of her pain and my caring for her I am exhausted. I can't go on any longer.

"You need a good cry," she says, "not for me but for yourself, for your own struggles."

She draws me close, embraces me, strokes my head and back. I have a huge lump in my throat, can hardly breathe. Then it releases, a great flood of tears, cries and groans, grief and despair. I feel myself dissolving in my tears.

And my tears seem to give her energy. Earlier she was feeling tired and listless but for the rest of the evening she is more alive and energised.

In the middle of all this process the world hears my cry for help. Brenda offers to come once a week to clean the house for us. Gerda and Leslie, friends from the Process Work group, bring over a casserole for us. Jo has been round to cook meals. Val and Syd come to give reiki.

Later in the month Amanda feels better, gets up and we go for a short walk. She is so delighted to be out in nature again, to see the autumn trees and crunch the leaves beneath her feet. In the evening we get the sewing machine out and do a little more on the curtain making which we still have not finished. It's a joy to work creatively together.

16

The weeks pass and Amanda feels well enough to go to a Process Work seminar in Oxford that is to explore how to live a meaningful life while dealing with difficult symptoms. It's spread over five days so we drive over there daily and come home in the evenings. She finds it inspiring but is often tired and has to rest whenever possible. There are people there with all kinds of illness and the therapists Max and Jytte help them explore and unfold some of the mysterious hidden wisdom that lies within our bodies in dealing with our symptoms. We both feel encouraged by the sense that we are not alone in dealing with huge problems.

Amanda shares her experiences with the group and works with Max. He helps her discover and get in touch with a powerful creative energy that lurks beneath her Leukaemia. Later she tells me she had a feeling of something opening up inside her. She makes a drawing of a bird in flight with flaming wings which she calls her fire-bird. It is an inspiring image of energy for her writing and creative work. At the end of the seminar she asks Max to be her therapist over the coming time, and he agrees to help her, over the phone if he is not available in person.

I too work with Max. I come to see that Leukaemia is a powerful energy for change. It is an energy with its own agenda, and not concerned whether humans live or die. It simply demands that we find ways to respond to it. We cannot opt to ignore it. My response is to open my heart to the mysteries of love and my mind to the mysteries of life. I feel a new space opening inside me where I can grow.

Some intuition tells me I should go to another seminar in Oxford for two more days, this time on working with people who are in a coma. I learn ways to relate and communicate with people who are unconscious and may not be able to see or hear me. Working in pairs we take turns to act the role of the carer and the person in a coma. I sit watching the breathing and movements of my partner and discover that seemingly meaningless actions, such as a sudden deeper breath, a twitch of the arm, actually reveal that the person is still there and conscious of the world around. Being present in heart and soul beside an unresponsive body is a new way of relating.

I am told that someone in a coma may still be able to hear what people are saying and doing. I lie down and act as if I am in a coma myself, imagining myself unable to see or move and unable to speak or tell others I am still alive and present. I find it terrifying. And it is a great comfort to know that I have a partner out there who is looking out for me and explaining what is going on. I can barely move at all and the only way I can express anything is with little jerks of my legs and twitches of my eyes. It helps when my 'carer' responds positively to these, either with a gentle touch or some loving words.

As a result of these seminars I feel stronger and better prepared to deal with whatever comes up for us in the future. I may need to use some of this if Amanda gets much worse.

17

Early December is full of pain and sickness. Amanda is despairing, "I think I don't have long to live. I need to make a will, sort things out and put my affairs in order."

I feel a deep emptiness; my world is coming to an end. I am afraid I will lose my mind, go insane and not be able to return to myself. At David and Katy's house I let go and cry. Open hearted, they hear my pain. They don't tell me it will all be OK, don't try to fix it. They give me the gift of their attention.

Jean Claude says, "Lose yourself, let yourself go crazy and see what comes afterwards. It's only by making space in yourself that there becomes room for something new."

Amanda is wondering about other forms of healing. We make an appointment to see Stephen Turoff, a psychic surgeon. We drive out to Colchester and find a porta-cabin where he works beside a bleak roundabout not far from the motorway. A notice on the door says, 'This is spiritual healing. Don't stop taking your medication.' Despite the setting there is a real sense of peace around him. Amanda lies on the couch and he puts his hands on her head and shoulders, asking God for healing while he makes the movements of removing something from her body. I can't help feeling a bit sceptical watching him as he performs his 'surgery'. On our way home we talk of the experience and agree that while he may not have resolved her physical problems we both feel we have been touched somehow, are more accepting of the truth that she might die soon.

Once we are back home again I remind her we have a three-day clown meeting and theatre performance in Harlow near London. I want to go and ask her how she feels about it.

"It would be good for you to go," she replies, "I'm not well enough to do it just now, and I can get friends to come and stay. But can we think of going somewhere warm on holiday after Christmas?"

Again that sinking feeling and aching heart. I say, "Yes that's a good idea." But inside I feel fear. Fear that she may not ever be able to make a big journey like that again.

It's a relief to get away from the sick room, to get fully involved in the work of preparing our theatre performance. I love so much of what is involved: stage preparation, the lighting, costumes, and makeup. I love being on stage and the sense of togetherness it all generates. Regular calls back home keep me in touch with Amanda. She has a friend staying and sounds well. She hears the energy in my voice and is pleased I am doing what I want and enjoying myself.

Christmas is a family time; we stay with Amanda's mum and dad, see friends and other relatives. She is feeling okay.

But not for long. Just before New Year we drive to the hospital through a snowstorm and learn that her blood counts are worse than ever. They increase the medication.

"You know I've struggled with leukaemia for so long, I've had enough and feel ready to let go. I need to prepare myself for that."

I wonder what is coming next.

"I love you hugely, want to do lots of things together, but I also need to be on my own more. I need time alone to do what I need to get done. I am having such difficulty sleeping at night I think I would do better if I slept alone in my bed."

I know she is being honest, but I can't help feeling rejected. So much of the past months we have been very close together, and now I am not sure what to do. I've got into the habit of togetherness, and in that warm embrace I have again lost track of my individual self and my journey. Sharing a bed and cuddling together is such an essential and lovely part of our relationship. But I understand her need and move out into the other bedroom.

Actually I sleep better and surprisingly don't worry about her, but I still feel rejected.

Though she is often in pain we are quite active. We celebrate the New Year together with a little ceremony beside the fire. We visit Didier and Carola in London. Val and Syd come for supper and we have a reiki sharing session. I drive her to Colchester again to see Stephen Turoff. As before he helps us in subtle ways, so we both feel more at peace with life. We also wonder at his parting words when he turned to me and said, "When are you going to write your book?" We are both surprised as Amanda is the writer and I have no intention of writing anything.

Doing so much driving is wearing me out. The journey to Oxford takes forty-five minutes each way, and this week we have to go for a check-up on Monday, for a blood transfusion on Tuesday and to see the dentist on Wednesday. I am always driving. I spend ages looking for parking spaces, and then hours sitting in waiting rooms, and I'm getting very fed up with it. I know I can't change the fact that I have to drive but perhaps I can change the way I think and feel about it. Instead of seeing it as a nuisance I decide to make each journey a pleasure in its own right. I begin to practice breathing awareness while I drive and consciously take notice of whatever I see. I use the radio and cassette player more intelligently. I practice meditation in the waiting rooms and make sure I have either inspiring or entertaining books with me so that I have something good to read.

I often go back to 'Who Dies?' by Steven Levine. It helps me be more open to the mystery of dying. It reminds me I am not in charge of things, that I need to be open minded and flexible, listen to intuition and live life as it comes. My meditation practice helps still my disturbing thoughts.

Then one afternoon Amanda gets terrible tooth pains and is crying out, but refuses to call the dentist. I curl up and wince at her cries. Again there's nothing I can do or say and she doesn't want me in the room. I sit downstairs trying to distract myself with the television. I ring David for a chat but a few minutes later Amanda calls out from upstairs that she is desperate to phone the dentist so I hang up. But now it's too late for an appointment, even with an emergency dentist. She is weeping with pain, asks me to find the painkillers but they will take forty-five minutes to have any effect. I sit beside her and she complains I am stopping her from getting up.

She's cold and I help her put a shawl on. She wants to be left alone. I go downstairs but can still hear her sobbing with pain. I feel sad, miserable, helpless and don't know what to do with myself. It is unbearable.

Later, when the painkillers have done their work, we talk. "The pain was so intense, I was feeling vicious, like a feral cat," She said. "I wanted to scratch and bite. And at the same time I wanted to be looked after, touched in exactly the right way. I need your support and feel so guilty about asking so much of you."

The drugs make her drowsy and she falls asleep early. Unexpectedly I have the evening to myself. I am not used to time to myself and don't know what to do. Is this a foretaste of what is to come?

18

Soon after New Year Amanda gets in touch with Katherine House Hospice to find out more about them and what they do. They invite us to visit and have a look around.

"I can't believe I'm doing this," she says, "It's like an admission that I am getting near the end. It's so unreal."

Katherine House is just two miles up the road, a modern building on a lane away from the main road. The nurse is warm and welcoming, and shows us the various bedrooms, common rooms and dining room. It is calm and peaceful, such a contrast to all the hospitals we have known. She tells us they are there to support people all through their illness, not just for the last few days of their lives, and talks about the various alternative therapies they offer. I soon find tears of relief flowing down my cheeks. Here are people who will really help and support us. I can see Amanda is taking it all in, and sense that she feels good here too.

We meet the Macmillan nurse who talks about palliative care, and how their aim is to make illness as much of a pain free experience as possible. This is the first time we have had a serious discussion about pain management. It is an unexpected relief to be talking just about how to make her life more enjoyable rather than focussing on how to carry on the fight with leukaemia. She suggests Amanda should try taking a low dose of morphine on a regular basis, which would help relieve the pains she's been experiencing. She agrees to give it a try.

Amanda is relaxing. "I am beginning to realise that I can stop fighting and just let things be."

Afterwards we walk around the garden and sit on one of outdoor seats, feeling the winter sun warming our faces. Even in early January this is a pleasant place to be.

She starts taking the morphine, has more visits with the nurse to get the dosage right, but after a week or so decides not to continue with it.

"It does work, eases the pain, but I don't like the feeling that my mind is somehow affected. I don't want to be permanently sedated. I can cope with some pain, and I want to retain my full consciousness. And anyway quite often the pain is not from my illness but from the discomfort of lying in bed so much."

On fine days Amanda and I go out for a walk in the mild sunshine. She can manage a few hundred yards if she takes my arm and we go really slowly. At home she does a little cooking and clearing up, and if she has the energy does some writing. The rest of the day she sits in an armchair with her feet up reading, watching television and talking to friends on the phone. Other days we might go for a drive or visit friends for a break.

I am helping her sort out her clown photos and putting them into an album.

"Who will get to see this?" she wonders. "It makes me think of all the things I love that I may never get to do again: clowning, singing, writing, walking in the woods, hanging out with friends, listening to music, cooking nice meals."

We share our sadness.

Wonderful Brenda still comes to clean the house each week, and Amanda's dad, who is a good cook, has prepared several meals for us to put in the freezer. He has also offered to pay our gas and electricity bills which have gone up so much because she suffers terribly from the cold. Another friend, Jenny, comes to visit and brings us lunch. Carola comes to visit and the three of us do a little clown improvisation together. It's good to feel all their support.

In my session with Jean Claude, he says I need to be more aware of my body's natural energy. I need to move and dance more often to reconnect with my physical being.

Visiting the hospice does not mean we have given up on the hospital. Amanda has agreed with the doctors she should have another round of chemotherapy. After the first session she feels bright and cheerful and we go out for supper in a restaurant and have a lovely evening. The next morning she feels awful and wonders if it was really worth it. I hope she means the chemo, not the meal out.

One of the things I have to deal with is the phone calls from friends. They ring up and the first thing they say is, "How is

Amanda?" I don't know how to answer. What should I tell them? Do they want to know that she has had injections, chemotherapy, has been sick, is feeling fed up and depressed? Do I say 'not very strong but in good spirits', or simply 'as good as can be expected'? Some of them tell me they want to hear it from me as they think I will describe the situation more honestly than she might.

Amanda doesn't like so much attention being focused on her health.

"I feel as if I've become an object of curiosity for everyone. They just see me as a sick person and forget that I am also a living human being with hopes and fears and an intelligent mind. All this talk about illness creates a bad atmosphere, makes it feel as if we are living in a house of sickness, and then it's even harder for me get away from the sense of always being ill."

Later that month Amanda has friends to stay while I go to Edinburgh for a two day Process Work seminar. The workshop gives me space to just unwind and helps me to look more closely at how I am in our relationship. I become more aware of how strong my need for intimacy is, and how this comes into conflict with my need to be free and independent. I know that Amanda has similar issues, and that is why we struggle together at times.

After all the travelling I'm happy to come back home, but things are difficult between us and we start to have arguments.

"I don't feel at all nice and friendly," she says. "I feel hard and unpleasant, all prickly. I've had enough. I feel trapped.

Trapped by my illness, trapped in this house and trapped in our relationship. I want to get out of it all. I want to live separately, to be freer, to be more myself."

At once I feel both angry and rejected. But I manage not to react negatively, not to say I am fed up and have had enough as well. I make an effort to see how we can find a way forward.

"I know you feel trapped and want freedom. Me too. We're really stuck, and we seem to have lost our closeness and intimacy at the same time. What can we do to make things work better?"

"There probably isn't anything either of us can do. It helps just to know you understand."

"I need to say a bit more," I add. "I sometimes feel you take me for granted, forget how much I do to support you. It's me who looks after you when you are in pain, ferries you here and there in the car and who pays the rent and the bills. I need more of a sense of being valued in this relationship."

"I'm sorry," she replied. "I may not show it all the time but I really do appreciate you and everything you do for me."

We agree to leave it there. Actually over the following days we get closer again, and have some lovely time together. Our emotional ups and downs are a regular feature of our lives. Our closeness and warmth brings out the sadness and poignancy of our situation.

Today, unexpectedly, she is feeling much better, well enough to drive the car, and has gone off to visit Val, do some shopping and go for a walk. I feel relieved and begin to imagine she will go on feeling well. I wonder what has brought about such an effect, it could be the homeopathy, acupuncture, spiritual healing or else the chemotherapy. It's impossible to know.

19

As so often the future comes unexpectedly.

We are at the hospital for a routine check-up, in the consultant's office. He has several sheets of paper in his hands.

"I'm afraid the results of the tests this time show that your condition is getting worse. These are your blood counts, and you can see they are lower than ever." He shows us a page giving dates and figures. "You are getting weaker and I can't see that things are going to improve much."

He looks directly at Amanda and goes on, "I think it's time for you to do whatever is most important in your life, as that may not be possible for much longer."

This feels like a death sentence, so much at odds with how she feels. Do we believe it? We talk about miracles and unexpected healing, wanting to believe in them. We know that hope itself is a powerful and positive force, after all the hospital is basing its opinion on statistical evidence, and there are always exceptions. We don't want to give in to despair because they say it is inevitable, nor do we want to be naive and get lost in some fantasy that the situation is not serious.

What does she want to do? Finish the book she is writing? Go for a holiday? Or simply carry on as usual? It seems rather short notice for such big decisions.

"Actually," she says, "I've been trying to do what is important for many years. Leukaemia taught me that."

"Oh, yes," I reply. "I wasn't thinking."

"So, I want to carry on as we are, sometimes together, sometimes apart. I want to spend time with my friends and doing the things I enjoy. There isn't any particular great thing that I need to do."

"In a sense," she continues, "I've been lucky in having such a teacher. We're all going to die sometime, and my 'luck' is to have all this warning that it is going to happen in the not too distant future. I haven't been able to live with some fantasy that I will live for ever. It's just made more poignant by the fact that I am still young."

This all makes sense to me. And then I wonder about myself. What do I want to do during this time? I am desperately sad that she might die soon and can't bear to think about what she might have to go through. Of course I want to be close to her as much as possible and make her life as easy as I can but I'm afraid of the future, of her dying. How will I cope with her suffering and how I will survive after she has gone? And when I'm not having those thoughts and feelings I want to do ordinary things such as meeting up with my clown friends and studying Process Work. And I need to earn some money.

In the night she cries. "I don't want to die. I don't want to die. I want to go on living. I am so envious of you because you will go on doing things, seeing friends, living life, and I won't do any of that."

I sit with her and listen. My heart aches.

In the morning she is calmer. She wants to talk about her funeral.

I have to make a mental effort to follow her, to make myself think about it, this unimaginable event.

"Who is the funeral for?" She asks. "Is it for me or for the people who will be there? Will I be there in some way and be involved in what happens?"

"I guess it's for both you and the others. You might be up there watching."

"Hmmm," she grimaces, "maybe."

I realise we have never actually talked about what happens after someone dies. Neither of us believes in an afterlife, but coming back for another life in a different form seems more possible. But it's not something we hold on to, or use for comfort.

"No church service please. Perhaps a village hall. I want music from Adiemus and for us to sing The Lord is my Shepherd. Perhaps some good rock music too. And spread my ashes in Wales, on the mountain where I once felt so wild and free."

"Okay," I say, "but can we talk about this another time. I can't face thinking about it now."

It's the not knowing that is so difficult. Is she really going to die soon? Should she accept her fate and allow things to take their course? Or should she put more energy into looking for treatments, homeopathy, shamanic healing and others? If you accept that you will die soon does that somehow make it more likely to happen? Do you get to a stage where you just let go?

I feel annoyed that there is no-one to guide us through it all, no-one to tell us how others have found their way through it in the past. After all people have been dying for millennia and yet we still don't know how to deal with it. Death and dying is treated as something rare and unpleasant, never to be looked at and discussed. We really should have answers. Dying is such a significant part of living and it comes to all of us, yet it always comes as a surprise, something we are not ready for.

Then I come across a chapter in 'The Tibetan Book of Living and Dying' where I find a fascinating detailed description of what happens in the process of dying, and what the spirit goes through on its way to rebirth. It gives me unexpected insights into the time immediately before death and afterwards. I am not a Buddhist, but I find this book really helpful.

So we go on as best we can, and amidst it all I still do the cooking, washing up, driving, shopping and laundry.

20

Amanda has a high temperature and feels terrible so we drive to hospital.

"I feel utterly helpless," she says at the entrance, "like a little child being sent off to boarding school. I am afraid I'll never come out of here again."

She sees the registrar who tells her she has an infection and will need to stay in for a few days to clear it up with intravenous drugs.

"Just as I feared."

We have two hours to wait before the consultant is free. When we do get to him he is looking serious.

"I'm sorry I have to say this to you, though I expect you've already realised it." He pauses. "There is really nothing more we can do about your leukaemia."

"Hmmm. And how much longer does that mean I have?"

"Probably only a few weeks."

I am so filled with sadness that I don't hear any more of the conversation. Later Amanda says she was not surprised, she had not thought the chemo was anything other than a temporary relief.

While waiting for the hospital to arrange a bed we talk about how to live the coming weeks.

"What do we say to people?" I ask, "Do we tell them you don't have much longer?"

"I don't want you to tell everyone. I'm afraid it could somehow generate a negative energy that would accelerate my dying. But," she goes on, "we have to be honest. Perhaps not too blunt. It depends who you are talking to. I'm afraid there will be a sudden surge of sympathy and then a whole crowd of visitors. I don't want that."

"OK. We'll have to try to manage that."

I give her a gentle massage, feeling what a joy it is to touch her in this way, wanting to go on for a long time so I will be able to remember it in the future. I have to make an effort to stay in the present, living and experiencing life as it is right now, and not drift off into the future.

Over the next days she has visitors in hospital and I take time to go out and be with my friends. Mostly I just cry as I tell them how my life is. They are gentle and warm with me, just being there and listening, not trying to tell me things will be all right.

Amanda starts to make her will, deciding what to do with her favourite belongings.

I read more of Who Dies? and feel supported and uplifted.

21

I am at home, alone, having spent the afternoon with her in hospital. I don't know what to do with myself. I take out my journal to try and find a way to express my feelings in writing. Each step along this path is so painful. It seems I have to experience all this with such intensity, to suffer the terrible slow journey, step by step, till the end.

All that afternoon
We were so tender and open
Loving and vulnerable
Knowing yet not believing
In the truth of what was happening

A pool of tenderness
Gathered behind my eyes
Held from overflowing
By the clarity of your presence.

22

It's bitterly cold, and wet. Amanda is still in hospital.

I am at David and Katy's house, this place where our journey began and where I have returned so often.

The phone rings.

"The doctor says I only have a week to live."

"I'll be there soon."

I walk into the ward and see her sitting up in her bed. We hold each other, sharing, crying and trying to work out what to do next.

"I always knew I would get to this stage, but never expected it to feel like this. And I don't suppose a temporary cure, a respite of six months, would really change anything."

I don't want to go on without her.

Thoughts come and go.

Who will water the flowers?

She won't ever see the daffodils I planted.

What shall I do with our new food processor?

There will be no-one to love and no-one to love me.

Am I just being selfish? What about her?

"They say I can go home today."

23

Back home together.

She is sleeping.

The slowest morning.

What do I do?

Waiting. For what?

I try to meditate, pray.

The sun is out and I sit in the garden. A blackbird hops up close and looks me in the eye. He understands.

The daffodil bulbs I planted are just sprouting.

24

We visit Katherine House again. We spend time talking with the hospice nurse about how they can help her. Either they will come and see her at home or she can come and stay in the hospice. We see the Macmillan nurse, the one who really understands pain management.

Amanda is very clear. "The most important thing for me is to be conscious. I want to live fully right up to the last moment; I want to be awake as I die. So I don't want any sort of drug that will cloud my mind."

"What happens if you are in a lot of pain?"

"If it gets so bad that I can't think clearly then maybe some painkiller would be helpful. But I am wary of morphine and how it changes the mind."

"We can control the drugs very precisely and I'll do my best to give you what you want."

I listen in awe. How can she be so real and thoughtful under these circumstances?

Afterwards we walk in the garden and talk about our situation.

"I am wondering whether to spend my last days here or at home. I have to decide where I want to die."

This is such strange territory. I am moved by the simple clarity of the way she talks about it. If it were me, I would choose home as it's more friendly and familiar.

Later that afternoon she says, "I think it might be best to go into the hospice. I feel it would be easier to detach from life there. There's too much, too many things, in the house here that I will want to hold on to."

I can understand. Dying means leaving everything you are familiar with, and it could be easier to leave by stages rather than all in one go. But I feel sad and hurt. It's as if she's choosing to leave me here as well. But I accept this is what is actually about to happen and that it is the most significant time in her life. It is also the most significant time in my life. I have to simply stay in the present moment and be a part of the process, to feel my feelings of pain and despair, and to help and support her in whatever way I can.

Back at home I see she is losing interest in normal daily life. It's up to me now to decide anything practical about the house. I seem to be crying all the time, tears in my eyes and a great lump in my throat. I feel heavy and strange, as if something is about to break.

25

"I'm sure now that going into the hospice will be the right thing, and I've decided I want to go in tomorrow."

"Okay. I will help you. Let's try and have a nice evening tonight."

With a heavy heart I make us supper of steamed vegetables and rice.

I read aloud from Who Dies?, the chapter about letting go.

We listen to some of Amajee's talks and Indian chants.

I give her reiki.

We are peaceful. We have come through storm and chaos to a place of calm acceptance.

"I have stopped fighting," she says, "I surrender."

"I feel more at ease now too. I know I'll be able to cope with whatever comes."

26

It's a sunny day. The world is bright and fresh.

She was awake in the night, angry that she has to go. Now she is calmer, more reflective.

"I still can't believe this is happening. It's so strange.

"We are running out of loo paper, but I suppose it's not my business any more. The bathroom mat needs washing, and it probably won't get done. My closest friends, Carola, Didier and Paula will be staying tonight and I won't be here."

She packs her overnight bag, carefully choosing clothes, books, a picture of Amma and things from the mantelpiece.

"This can't be true. Am I really going? Do I have to?"

I watch as she comes down the stairs, looking around, for the last time.

As she closes the front door behind her.

As she walks down the path and carefully shuts the gate.

As she gets in the car.

I start the engine.

27

She has a room to herself, pastel coloured walls and a window out onto the garden. She unpacks and puts her clothes away in the chest of drawers. We are served a light lunch in the dining area.

The nurses are always around and helpful but not intrusive and I see how well they will look after her. I feel an immense sense of relief that I can let go of the work of caring for her. I start crying. These tears are different, they are for me. I have born so much for so long, the strain has been immense, and now it is over. I am crying for myself, for all the struggles I have been through.

Afterwards I feel calm. I stop thinking of the past and the future and can simply be with Amanda as she goes into her dying process. She is right to come here. We put so much into making our home sweet and lovely, a place that held us gently as we lived our lives together. Now she has left it behind, along with all her clothes, possessions, interests and activities. There are no distractions here and that is how she wants it.

We sit peacefully. She is clear in her head, knows exactly what she wants now she is at this stage.

"I may be nearing the end," she says, "and I want you to know that while I never wanted to die of leukaemia, I would not want to have lived without it. Leukaemia has been my greatest guide and teacher, demanding that I wake up, grow up and become the person I truly am."

I am amazed that she can say these words in this situation.

"Now I want to be left on my own for a while, to follow my inner process. Will you come back this evening?"

I go back to the house. It's strange to walk up the familiar path to the front door. Everything looks the same and yet it's empty. I'm empty, yet full. My head is confused, can't take it all in, and it's as if my heart has stopped. I am in the space between the worlds, between life and death. The future is a mystery and I am pregnant with an unknown birth ahead of me.

I go round the house, into every room, absorbing its existence and its emptiness. I see the huge pot of marmite she bought a few days ago and wonder who will eat it now.

I go for a walk, wandering aimlessly through the woods, seeing the trees and seeing nothing. I am internal, filled with unfamiliar feelings that as yet have no form of expression.

I phone Jean Claude. He is attentive. "Stay in the present, be open hearted, don't try to work things out. Be true to yourself; find ways to express your feelings that don't disturb her. Stay in the Tao, in the flow. Don't fight it."

I find that helpful, to be reminded to simply be myself in the here and now, and that there is nothing else I need to do.

The answer machine shows twelve messages. I think I ought to reply and manage to make two calls.

Then it's evening, time to return to the hospice. She has arranged her things, created an altar with the picture of Amma, a shell, a starfish, a leaf, a piece of dried bark and a little vase of snowdrops. I fluff up her pillows, give her reiki and lightly massage her feet. Our togetherness is sweet, made poignant by the knowing that it will not last for long.

The nurses say they have a room for families where I can sleep if I want or I can stay in her room.

I choose to be with her.

28

A grey Monday morning, a storm is brewing. Amanda is sitting up in bed and I sit quietly beside her.

She has a phone session with Max, her psychotherapist, so I go for a walk. Afterwards she is relaxed and present, an air of grace emanating from her.

We are expecting visitors who will want to spend time with her.

"I'd like to see just one or two people at a time, and no emotional outbursts. I can't deal with other people's feelings any more."

Carola and Didier arrive, sweet and tender. Didier leads us in a Buddhist meditation. Paula arrives, a close and important friend of Amanda's, offering to stay if that will help. She is a lovely wise woman and I find her presence a huge support. Other friends come and go.

"It feels as if they have come to say goodbye. I don't need that now, it's too painful. Can you make sure others don't come with that in mind."

"I'll try to explain," I say. "Can you say what you do want from them?"

"Just to be with me, as we are, as we have been in the past. Just to feel our friendship. Not to make it a dramatic last farewell. And I would rather not see Teresa, she is too controlling and I am afraid she will try to take charge. I can't cope with that. Will you be my gatekeeper, my guardian? Will you look after those things?"

"OK," I know this could be difficult, but I accept that it's what she wants. "I'll ask Paula to help as well."

"Now I need some time alone, I need to just be by myself while I go into this. It's a journey I have to make alone and I feel very fearful, but it's what I need to do. I want to meditate and remain in the deepest part of my being. Can you make sure no-one disturbs me, not even you."

I understand and respect her wishes, but at the same time feel as if I've been dismissed. My mind and feelings are in conflict and I look for Paula to talk about it and help me to let it go.

I sit in the garden, peaceful again despite the fierce cold wind. All the stress is gone. She is no longer fighting leukaemia, the doctors are not working to keep her alive and I am not struggling to be her carer.

I am surrendering, letting life do what it needs to do. Like a river I am in the flow, following the Tao.

At night I curl up to sleep on the sofa beside her bed.

29

Another day dawns with a fierce gale roaring, blowing and buffeting the building. It seems the earth is responding to this passing of a soul.

Her room is decorated with flowers; candles shine brightly and the scent of incense fills the air. There is a feeling of peace and stillness, an air of delicate anticipation. A momentous event is unfolding and people are gathering to be witness.

Paula is still here and Lucy, another old friend of Amanda's, has come to stay. We meditate in silence in her room. We talk softly to each other, spend time with Amanda one to one.

The nurses come and go, remake her bed, change her clothes, monitor her pain and administer pills to keep her comfortable. I appreciate all their care and attention that make this all possible for Amanda and the rest of us.

I take a walk out alongside the lake and in the woods. The snowdrops are coming out.

I am pleased for Amanda that her friends are here, but I feel invaded. I find it hard to share her with these others who were not there to support her in all the last difficult months. I know they are her dearest friends, but I feel resentful and am jealous of her time. And to make it even harder, she wants to have plenty of time on her own.

I have to let go of all of this, I will need to learn to live without her soon enough. At least I have those precious hours of the night when we are together and can be close.

30

Wednesday morning and the gale is still raging outside.

Paula, Lucy and I chat and take turns to be with Amanda.

We, this little group of helpers, gather round the table for lunch and sit still for a minute in silence. At that moment the door to your room opens:

And you just appear
small and frail
in your blue dressing gown
walking erect
as if surprised at yourself
wondering that your legs
could still carry you.

It's your smile
that touches my heart

it holds some deep inner joy
and calm serenity.
You sit softly
in the armchair
so light
the cushions barely stir
beneath you.

Amongst the cards that come in the post is a CD of some klezmer music you had ordered. You ask me to put it on the player.

The fiddles start slow and mournful, then gradually quicken in rising excitement as the clarinet begins its swirling flight. You smile, light shining in your eyes as your fingers take the rhythm, your hands dance lightly in the air. I wonder if you, like me, recall a year ago in Devon on your birthday how you danced upon the tables, a wild gypsy woman with drumming and guitars.

Later you walk to the table
slow and careful
sure of your mind
unsure of your body
sit erect
eat a little
sip your water
say a few words

taking pleasure in every moment
of this simple gathering.

At last you rise
and leave
softly
as you came
walking away
down the corridor
to your room.

31

On Thursday we have phone calls from Theresa, Pam, Linda, Soraya, Rob, Val all wanting to come and visit. I am glad Paula and Ruth take some of the calls. How do you say, "Yes, she is really ill, and she might be dying, but she doesn't want you to come and visit." Most understand but Theresa is angry saying I am trying to shut her out.

Amanda's sister Ruth arrives with her friend Pete. She joins our little group of carers and takes time sitting with Amanda.

Then Lucy drops a bombshell, "Amanda wants me to sleep in her room tonight instead of you."

I am shocked, as if I have been punched in the stomach. Our nights together have been so sweet and precious. Now I feel hurt and rejected. But when I think about it I don't believe it's as simple as that. I don't think Amanda would have suggested such a thing, but I can't go and ask her.

I'm angry and have had enough, so much that I want to get away. I escape back to the house with Ruth and Pete, pour out all my rage, hurt, despair and exhaustion, like an angry lover who has been cruelly deserted. I let it all out and they hear me. And then it turns itself around and somehow we end up laughing uproariously. I feel better, freer to be myself, just as Jean Claude had recommended. In a strange way this has helped me in my process. It's the catalyst that helps me break out of the trance-like state of being the nice caretaker. I can be more truly myself, let go of everything, and then carry on doing what I need to do for Amanda.

Back in the hospice when I am with Amanda I stay calm and present. But out in the visitors' room, often with Pete, I let the grief and tears come out. He listens, helps me release all my feelings.

My throat is sore with sobs of despair. My eyes are red and painful. There is a pain in my heart and it gets more intense as the day goes on. It's a real physical pain and suddenly I am afraid. How much worse can it get? Is my heart going to burst? Can you die of a broken heart? Is that what's happening to me?

At last, exhausted, I lie down and fall asleep, feeling better when I wake.

I want to listen to klezmer music again, and there is an empty room I can use. I plug in the music player and turn the volume up. I move slowly with the rhythm. As it speeds up I move faster, more strongly, flowing and turning. Ever faster and wilder, spinning, leaping, into a wild and crazy beautiful dance that goes on and on. I seem to dance forever until I collapse exhausted on the floor, laughing and crying.

32

Early morning
and still the storm outside

In here you are restless
I sit by your bed
seeing and sharing
each breath
each move
each moan and cry of pain.

Your eyes open
and you smile.
"Do you think I am dying now?
are these my last days"
"Yes, I think so."
"Mmm"

You slip in and out of consciousness
making your journey
towards the centre of your being
from where you will finally leave.
Feeling your way
each time a little further
and coming back
as if reassuring yourself
that it's safe to go so far.

Once more you open your eyes
smile tenderly
and reach out to touch me.

Others come and go. We talk and share this loving care, we who have been chosen as companions on this road.

The nurses tend you lovingly, concerned for your pain and discomfort and they want to increase the medication. We talk about your wish to remain conscious and be free of distracting pain. I unhappily accept they may be right.

By the evening you are travelling further
and come back less
growing surer in your journey
trusting us to keep you safe

You go on
deep into your inner world
less concerned with us.
All through the night
into the dawn,
a mysterious time
beyond the measure of a clock

Your breath is so light
a sacred sigh
as the air slips softly
between your lips.

At last the wind has ceased. Dawn breaks
and the sun rises in extraordinary silence.
All is poised and attentive to the moment

Throughout that time stopped morning
we share our vigil
quiet and still
awed by the sound of your breath
as it grows from peaceful whisper
to a heavy rasping rhythm

we move in and out
slipping softly through the door
to eat and talk

on through the afternoon
in silent wonder
we sit
until on impulse
Ruth takes your had
and gives a squeeze
as if to say its all OK

And then you change
we are all aware its nearly done
this is the moment
you take three
deep
peaceful
breaths

and then no more

An awesome silence fills the room

No-one moves

I sense your consciousness

rising out of your body

and feel your presence in the room

with joy I realise you are still there

you have not ceased to exist

We are blessed to witness this

Time passes

people leave softly in ones and twos

and go back to the house

Each one has been deeply touched

our hearts are open

This is the gift we have each received

To have our hearts opened

This is the gift in Amanda's dying

We are expanded and released into a greater consciousness

33

After the funeral, the talk and the memories
family and friends depart
back to their normal lives

I am alone

I have no normal life

I come and go between realities
my inner world of heart and unseen presence
the outer world of people and events

There is no time, no time scale for this
waves of emotion wash through
I am wracked with grief and pain
longing and desire
loneliness and despair

I sit in the bay window
and watch the sunrise
the daffodils coming into flower
the magnolia opening its buds
blackbird song fills my ears
and the sun warms my face

There is nothing left of me
I have been through the flaming inferno
my human flesh has been burned away
and all that remains is my white skeleton
I am in a state of purity
of grace

I build an altar in our living room
your ashes in an urn, your photo
a piece of rock, some flowers
a candle and a bowl of water

I sit
in silence
sending love and good wishes
hoping they will help you
on your journey
honouring your transition
from life in a body
to being pure spirit

I feel your presence
and know that you live on

34

I continue in this state of timelessness for weeks

I take a bath
have breakfast
wait for the post

I sit in the garden
feel the heat of the sun
no thoughts
no need to talk
or put on my personality

But at night it is different

In the night I am vulnerable
Fear and loneliness constrict my heart
then rage and despair
rampage through my body
so I toss and turn relentlessly through the hours
And when I drift off into sleep
desire comes unexpectedly
disturbing my rest with wild erotic dreams
I am thrown helpless between
these outrageous powers
until deeper sleep releases me into oblivion

35

Six weeks have gone by and I am getting used to living alone.

I clean the house, do the laundry, go shopping as usual, but now it's just for myself. I used to do things as part of our loving relationship, in a sense I did them for her. Now it is simply what I have to do to live.

I am slowly sorting and clearing her belongings and her presence feels less intense. But still I trip over the unexpected. I had put some of her things down in the hall, ready to take to Oxfam. Later I come out of the kitchen and see her walking shoes by the front door. All my sense of loss returns in a flash, my heart jolts and tears fill my eyes.

One evening I put on a video borrowed from the library. I hadn't realised it was a film about loss, it was Shadowlands, about C S Lewis and his wife who was dying of cancer. As I watch it I cry and cry but somehow I know I need to see it. It seems I have more tears to release so I spread it over a few days, a bit at a time.

I still feel a stranger to the world, and I don't have a hold on life.

It is more as if life is holding me.

36

I wonder if it's time for me to get out into the world and be more active. In search of guidance I throw the I Ching and it directs me to hexagram 56 entitled Travelling. It says, 'you are travelling through the situation in hand. You will move on in time but don't try to make long term plans. Hold on to your integrity, it may become your lighthouse in this sea of the unknown.'

These words support me in staying where I am, not trying to achieve anything. It is still time to rest, recover and digest all I have been through, to let my experiences consolidate their effects on my psyche and allow those inner processes and transformations that are taking place to come to fulfilment. And I find the image of my integrity as a lighthouse is encouraging, meaning I can trust my deepest self and that it will be my guide in times to come.

Another day I am having doubts about the wisdom of the way I am going through this grief and I am given hexagram 48 called the Source. It speaks of 'the well, that deep, inexhaustible, divinely centred source of nourishment and meaning for humanity' and says that we need to return to this well to find fulfilment. Then it tells me that by putting my life in order now I will be able to contribute to the world more fully in the future. Again I feel reassured that what I am doing is right for me.

In another part of this hexagram I find an unexpected piece about relationships with others which says 'there are universal truths that bring certain individuals together.' That touches me, affirms what I had always thought, that our relationship was greater than either of us could understand.

37

Today I am relaxed and my mind is clear and sharp. I have been thinking about what we went through, trying to find an understanding of it all.

It's clear to me that your consciousness was not just snuffed out like a candle when you died. What I saw was that as you got closer to death you withdrew from the world and became more and more concentrated deep inside, until at last you were completely in your centre, with no connection to the rest of your body or what was outside it. From there you were able to slip over some boundary into another form of existence, leaving your inert body behind.

Afterwards I could sense your presence and help you through sending love and prayer. I also received help from you in the form of unexpected images and intuitions as well as strange coincidences in the world. It was a joy to realise this communication is a two way process.

I thought about my own processes, the peaceful daytime and the chaotic nights. I understand that these dark and shadowy aspects of my being are as much a part of me as the sensitive, meditative one who sits peacefully in the warmth of the sun. I am learning to live with all these different parts of and accept that this is what it means to be fully human.

What I don't know yet is how to live this out in the normal world.

38

It is three months now. I'm sorting out the rest of her possessions, what to keep and what to let go. I am returning to the world and having thoughts about the future. Jean Claude is running a residential creativity workshop in Norwich for a week, which appeals to me. I am thinking of going to India in the autumn.

Philip and I go to Great Missenden to run a weekend clowning workshop. It's lovely, flows effortlessly. My open and vulnerable feelings help others to be more open.

After a Fools Gold clowning weekend I spend the evening with Carola, talking about Amanda, death and clowning and how these are affecting all our lives. Carola's warmth and calm wisdom help me in my journey towards understanding and appreciation of all I have been given.

I miss Amanda and often find I am doing things the way that she would do them. I am more open-hearted, give more attention to the world around me, and am generally more sensitive. I take more care about how I cook and what I eat. Many of my old attitudes to life have gone and I am a fresher and more lively presence in the world. I have learned how to love.

I walk by the river, sit on the bank and think back over all I have been through, pondering on how it has changed me.

I remember the voice speaking to me in the night after Amanda had told me about her leukaemia. *This is your role for the coming years. To help her and see her through. And you will receive more than you give. You will be transformed. This is the spiritual journey you are offered.*

I know I have been transformed. I have been woken up and brought into consciousness. Like the river before me I know there are hidden depths and features; much is concealed beneath the surface.

But how do I take this unfamiliar self out into the world? I am still too raw and vulnerable, and don't know how to integrate it all with normal life.

39

June, and I drive to Wales with her ashes in the urn. On Saturday morning I meet with her sister and friends, ten of us on a mountainside near Aberystwyth. It's cold and windy so we create a ceremony indoors, standing together holding her memory in our hearts and minds.

We climb the mountain and make a circle around the urn while Paula says a prayer and each one of us takes a handful of the ashes.

As we turn to face the great valley below a fierce gust of wind whips the ashes from our hands and flings them out over the grass and rocks and into space. Through my tears I know she is there now, pleased we had brought her remains here, delighted to be free like the wind, ecstatic in this final release from her earthly body.

Later, after a walk through the woods we go indoors to dance and celebrate. That night Nikki has a vivid dream of a red dragon rising from the ashes in the urn.

40

My grieving process is moving on, I am further down the river, out of the rapids and in calmer waters where the current flows more smoothly.

Your presence is less intense. Like the air I breathe, you are always there but often I am not aware of you.

I no longer need to stay still and internal. I have grown a new skin that covers my raw and open heart and protects my vulnerable self, so I am able to meet the rough and tumble of daily life.

I am being inexorably pulled out into life in the world. My body needs food, my mind needs thought, my heart needs people. I'm ready for life, for action. My attention is on the future.

I book up for Jean Claude's creativity seminar.

A friend is organising a trip to an ashram in the Himalayas. I like the thought of travel and buy a copy of the Rough Guide to India.

Soon I will give my notice to leave this rented house.

I'm ready to step forward.

My future is waiting.

ACKNOWLEDGEMENTS

It has taken nearly twenty years for me to be able to write this book, to fully absorb all we went through. In the process I have re-read the journals I wrote at the time, and gone back in memory through those times of love, confusion, joy and pain. This work has often been moving and cathartic. I have laughed and cried my way through it all, and struggled to find ways to express what I recalled.

I am grateful to Michael Elsmere and the members of the memoir writing group he established in Kingsbridge who helped me to find my writing voice and develop my form of expression. Michael's sensitive facilitation, encouragement and feedback were vital to my ability to carry on. Other members of the group, Jean Mooney, Clare Pawley, Christine Cooke and Caroline Born, who are all gifted writers, kept me going with encouragement, creative suggestions and critical feedback.

I thank Wendy Watkins who patiently read my original manuscript and found ways to encourage me to rewrite in the many places I was confused or lost.

David Colbourne, Katy Jennison, Sarah Hobson, Edwyna Beaumont, Orna Ross and Peter Binns generously gave their time in reading and editing my work, helping me to discover finer ways to express myself.

I thank my wife Caroline Born for her acceptance of the work I was doing and her support and encouragement.

I thank too all those who were close and supportive during and after Amanda's illness, many of whom are mentioned in this book, and my apologies for omissions and errors that may have crept in without my realisation.

RESOURCES

Britain's National Health Service supported Amanda with its immense resources of medical knowledge and treatments, and played a major role in keeping her alive for so many years.

The Bristol Cancer Centre was fundamental in opening up her awareness to all the other approaches she could take towards her life threatening disease. It has gone through various changes and is now known as *Penny Brohn Cancer Care*, still based in Bristol.

Katherine House hospice near Banbury, and the hospice movement in general, provide a highly sensitive and supportive situation where people can receive wonderful on-going help and comfort in dealing with serious forms of illness at all stages and particularly in living the last days of their lives.

Macmillan nurses were very helpful in offering palliative care and making Amanda comfortable. They understand pain and administer pain relief sensitively and more effectively than many doctors seem able to do.

Acupuncture is part of the traditional Chinese approach to health. It works in a completely different way from western medicine, has a totally different understanding of the body, energy and health and offers treatments that may seem very strange to someone used to western approaches. I have had treatments with very positive outcomes where the medical profession was unable to help.

Homeopathy works in a way that defies all rational logic, and is often vilified by mainstream medical professionals. Its approaches are subtle, personal and mysterious. Opening my mind to homeopathy has broadened my understanding of what it means to be well.

The right psychotherapist is important for emotional and mental health. He or she can be an essential support through difficult times, quite different from that which can be offered by other practitioners, friends or family. They can act as a catalyst helping to bring about deeper and wiser understanding of the often strange processes life can take us into.

Meditation helps still the mind and bring you back to your essential self. It's good to make it a daily habit.

Spiritual healing can bring comfort and relief and can have a profound effect on your psyche.

Amma, full name Mata Amritanandamayi Devi is a Hindhu holy person, an Avatar, who welcomes people of all nations. She has the Amritapuri ashram in Kerala, India and provides help for the poor in the form of homes, schools and hospitals and more.

Reiki is a hands on form of spiritual healing. After a short training you can offer this to friends and family. It simply involves sitting quietly with the other person with your hands placed gently on whatever part of the body is affected. It brings comfort and relief to the sufferer.

Humanistic Psychology takes the approach that we were all perfect beings at birth and that it is our subsequent experiences that have led us to grow and develop the way we have. It offers many different therapeutic processes to help resolve deep personal issues and find our way towards living a more fulfilling life. It contrasts with Clinical Psychology which has a more objective approach.

Co-counselling involves learning a set of techniques that open you to your deeper emotional life and help resolve your real life issues. In a co-counselling session you take turns with another co-counsellor to be the client and the counsellor, so there is no money involved and no authority figures to deal with. Co-Counselling International (CCI) offers short courses where you learn the techniques. After training you are responsible for your own process, and choose which co-counsellors you want to work with.

Process Orientated Psychology, often known as Process Work, is a comprehensive psychological approach developed by Arnold Mindell out of a combination of Jungian thought, quantum mechanics, intuitive processes and more. It identifies and works with the deeper levels of meaning that are expressed in our diverse and often incomprehensible experiences.

The Sacred Art of Clowning was developed by Lex van Someren, a perceptive teacher who ran trainings in it in the early 1990s. It helped to develop spontaneity, intuition and subtle awareness that may be helpful in dealing with unpredictable situations. He also taught skills for street and theatre performance. It is no longer offered in its original form, but people who worked with him have developed the work further in their own ways.

Fools Gold was a small group of clowns who had trained

with Lex and went on to work together in the late 1990s. I was a member and together we ran workshops and gave performances in schools, hospitals, and hospice as well as in businesses and theatres.

The I Ching is a system from ancient China used to explore the meaning of human life and affairs. By following a means of divination you are directed to one of the many pages of wisdom which offer fresh insight into your situation. I used the workbook put together by R L Wing.

Dreams have often brought me important understandings. It can be hard to make sense of vivid night-time dreams and I first learned to interpret them through Robert Johnson's book 'Inner Work'. Since then psychotherapists and Process Workers have helped me understand them further.

Change and variety is important for people with illness, to maintain a sense of well being and an interest in life. Time off for carers is essential to allow an opportunity to refresh and recharge one's energy and to feel 'normal' for a while.

Friends and family can bring warmth and loving presence and can offer help in whatever ways they are able. Illness can be a lonely time, no-one else is having your experience.

BOOKS THAT WERE HELPFUL

Who Dies? by Steven Levine

The Tibetan Book of Living and Dying by Sogyal Rinpoche

Grace and Grit by Ken Wilber

Coma, the Dreambody Near Death, by Arnold Mindell

A Path with Heart by Jack Kornfield

Lightning Source UK Ltd.
Milton Keynes UK
UKOW02f1501291116
288799UK00004B/156/P